A Beginner's Guid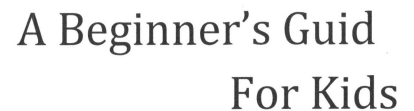
For Kids

50 Recipes That Kids Will Love

By

Sharon Daniels

Legal Disclaimers and Notices

Congratulations! You've just taking the first step in learning how to get your child to start a healthy, beneficial, and delicious juicing lifestyle.

Juicing is by far one of the easiest ways to get kids to meet their daily fruit and veggies requirements. Taking it one step further, you can add nuts, seeds, and grains for protein, or turn the juice into a smoothie using nonfat milk or yogurt for your child's daily dairy.

Juicing is the secret to getting those picky eaters and stubborn food-tossers the nourishment they need. We as parents know that getting your kids to eat enough fruits and vegetables can be stressful even at the best of times. Often, it's easier to get kids to eat fruit than vegetables, but even then, the amount of fruit they are usually willing to eat is not enough to meet the suggested daily servings. Juicing offers you a quick and delicious way to fill your little ones with the nutrition they need. Best of all, it's a fun way of getting their fruit and veggies that they won't be able to get enough of.

Consider this. If you make your child a raw juice made of beetroot, broccoli, and coconut juice, chances are they will drink the juice because it tastes yummy or because it is a cool color. Now try giving them bowl of beets and broccoli.

With my kids, it all goes downhill from there.

On the other hand, they actually enjoy the juice I described above because of the stellar difference in presentation.

That right there is the beauty of juicing. You can easily fulfill your child's daily fruit and veggie servings with one to two juices or green smoothies a day – and your child will be none the wiser!

Chances are you will be pleasantly surprised over how quickly your children will adapt to a

• • •

juicing regimen. You may notice that within a short while they will appear more evenly tempered, behave a bit better, sleep more soundly, and eat larger helpings at meals. You might even see an improvement in their schoolwork or after-school activities. All of these benefits come from the healing and mind-boosting properties of natural fruit and vegetable juices.

There is one decision that I believe is something that should be determined before introducing your kids to their new juicing regimen. Should you or should you not include your children in the making of the juices?

 Knowing your own child, is it wise to inform them about the ingredients in the juices – in other words, should you tell *your* child that they are drinking a cup full of fresh fruits and veggies? Would your child refuse to drink the juices if they knew? This is actually a very important decision to consider. You want your child to know, appreciate, and understand what they are eating and the benefits that come from consuming fresh produce – at the same time, you do not want to run the risk of them shutting down against the idea of juicing.

With many kids, just knowing that there are vegetables in something is enough to make them swear the food source off altogether. Kids are more likely to drink juices and smoothies made out of fresh fruits and vegetables than they are to eat the fruits and vegetables whole. They pick out their favorite foods based solely on the way they look and taste. They do not consider the nutritional value.

Of course, in a perfect world, your children would be helping you create the juices. They would recognize the ingredients, the benefits, and understand why the different fruits and vegetables are so good for them. However, this is not a perfect world, and most children would go down kicking and screaming, refusing to drink raw juices if they really knew that the juices were jammed full of fresh fruits and greens.

We, as parents, need to pick and choose our battles, and I for one would rather my children drink the raw juice because they liked the taste or the color as opposed to pushing them to learn and acknowledge the specifics of what they are consuming and why they are consuming it. For older children, this isn't so much of a problem – many of them enjoy learning the about the ingredients and experimenting with different fruits and vegetables. However, with younger children, tread lightly – you don't want to risk the chance of your kids refusing to drink the juices simply because they know the ingredients.

Throughout this book, you will discover simple juicing methods that will make introducing your kids to the juicing lifestyle safe and fun. **Kids are quick learners, which should make incorporating more healthy foods and less junk foods into their diets go smoothly. Later, I'll show you some tips...**

While introducing your child to the raw juicing regimen, it is important that you operate on a whole foods diet. Briefly, I'll discuss what this diet entails and why it is important to combine the diet with your child's juicing regimen.

Remember, many children aren't used to consuming their suggested daily requirements of fruits and veggies, so for the first week or two you may notice that your child begins experiencing bouts of gas, diarrhea, odd colored stools, constipation, minor weight loss, stomachache – this is all normal, and to be expected. You are prepping their little bodies to adapt to the larger consumption of fresh fruits and vegetables.

The whole foods diet will help prevent and reduce the severity of the above symptoms. It is therefore important to stick with the whole foods diet for as long as your child is juicing, or at least until their bodies adjust completely to the change in diet.

Make sure to ease them into the juicing and whole foods diet, especially if their usual diet contains not-so-healthy food choices like cheeseburgers and ice cream. If your child is not used to eating any fruits and vegetables, their symptoms may be more noticeable and last longer, so take baby steps. Work daily by replacing one snack with a juice or one meal with a whole foods meal. You don't want to push too much too soon – this will leave your child feeling bloated and yucky, which could discourage them from wanting to consume more of their juicing/whole food regimen.

As always, only you truly know your child and if you believe your child is having a harder than normal time digesting the fruits and vegetables or if any of the above symptoms last – without pause - for a period of more than two weeks, then it would be wise to schedule an appointment to meet with your pediatrician. Many times there are solutions that your doctor can offer your child that will allow their body to better tolerate the fruits and vegetables.

Above all, it's important to remember that children's bodies are different from our own and therefore digest certain foods differently. Use the recipes in this book to give you an idea of proper ingredient amounts for a child's digestive system. Before long, you will be an expert in knowing what your child can safely digest and you can begin experimenting with and creating your own recipes.

Now on your mark, parents! Get ready to introduce the kiddies to a nutritious, delicious lifestyle that will carry its benefits through their childhood and beyond.

Above all, remember to keep it fun! Have fun experimenting with different recipes and ingredients. If your child sees you having fun, then they in turn will view the experience as a fun one as well. You want your kids to view their juicing regimen as a treat; one they will eventually enjoy creating as much as they will love consuming!

TABLE OF CONTENTS

PART 1: INTRODUCING YOUR CHILD TO A JUICING LIFESTYLE

PART 1

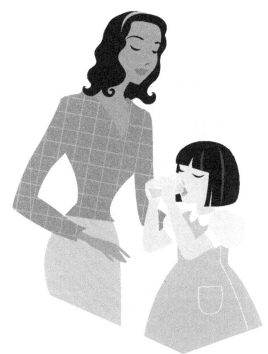

INTRODUCING YOUR CHILD TO A JUICING LIFESTYLE

CHAPTER 1: WHY IT'S IMPORTANT

Why Juicing is the Answer:

As parents, we know that a well-balanced diet is important for our children. A diet full of whole grains, dairy, meat, and of course fruits and vegetables plays a vital role in the overall growth and development of our children. However, realizing this doesn't make it any easier to impart it to our kids. If you've ever had a plate of broccoli thrown back at you by your three year-old, you understand why it's not so simple.

Kids like what kids like. They like cheeseburgers, spaghetti and meatballs, chicken nuggets, ice cream, and all those foods that not only contribute to obesity, but also do little to spur mental growth. Frankly, it's a win if we can get our kids to eat toaster waffles made with whole grain instead of the regular toaster waffles.

Getting our kids to eat healthy can be one of the hardest battles we face as parents, especially when we are fighting against all of the "fun" foods and sweets that kids like to eat. This is why juicing is a miracle in the making for many parents.

Kids love juice and smoothies. Not only that, but they're also so simple to make! Kids and parents alike are often on the go, which means that it can be difficult to eat a well-balanced diet throughout the day. (Don't get me started on the stuff they feed our kids in the school cafeteria.) So, being able to hand your kids a raw juice to drink on the way to soccer practice or piano lessons is something that they will love and you can feel good about. No need to tell them that they just drank two cups of spinach and carrots!

Now, there are kids out there who love fruits and veggies – they just can't get enough of them. For these parents, getting their kids to eat produce is as easy as putting it on a plate in front of them. To these parents – we applaud you! We only wish we knew your secret. It's these parents who can easily involve their kids in the juice making process since they won't flee the scene at the sight of a zucchini. For the rest of us, with our reluctant children – juicing is the perfect solution to our problems.

Juicing is the answer to getting our kids to eat the proper amount of fruits and veggies their bodies need to grow strong and healthy. Juicing can also help with many of the additional nutrition battles we have with our children. For example:

Problem: Your 5 year-old son REFUSES to drink milk, unless it's chocolate. You know he needs it to grow, but he looks at milk as if it's the enemy.

Juicing Solution: Turn the juice into a smoothie by adding 1 cup of nonfat milk *or* a ½ cup low-fat, fruit-flavored yogurt, and ice. Your son will love it! Do this a couple times per day to meet his daily dairy needs.

Problem: Your 13 year-old daughter comes home from school one day and swears that she is now a vegetarian. She insists that there is no way she will ever eat meat again. You know that she needs protein to grow.

Juicing Solution: Mix the juice with some nuts, seeds, or a scoop or two of protein powder. You can easily fulfill her daily protein requirements this way. In addition, fresh greens such as raw spinach are loaded with protein. Just by adding an extra ½ cup of raw baby spinach to her juice, you will boost your daughter's protein intake.

⌐ ⌐ ⌐ ⌐ ⌐ ⌐ ⌐ ⌐ ⌐ ⌐ ⌐ ⌐ ⌐ ⌐ ⌐

Problem: Your 7 year-old daughter refuses to eat any type of whole wheat or whole grains because she doesn't like the brownish color. You have tried everything, including trying to trick her with whole grain white bread and whole grain pasta, but somehow, she sees right through it every time and won't eat one bite.

Juicing Solution: Make her a green smoothie, but blend in with the fruit/veggies, a couple teaspoons of wheat germ, flax seed, and half to a whole banana to disguise the taste! She will love it, and won't be able to catch you this time!

How Juicing Benefits Your Little Ones:

Juicing provides children with a wide array of excellent benefits. Not only does juicing help with the physical and mental growth and development of our kids, but it also helps keep them energized and enthusiastic. It helps them to focus in school and events, it helps with overall coordination and vitality, and so much more! The benefits that come from putting your child on a juicing regimen are virtually limitless. Take a look below at some of the major benefits provided by a regular juicing diet:

Vitamins and Minerals:

Juicing helps provide our children with a wide assortment of vitamins and minerals that are perfect for their growing bodies. These vitamins and minerals help in numerous ways, some of which include:

- Strong Bones
- Strong, Healthy Teeth
- Healthy Hair and Skin
- Growth and Development (Mental and Physical)
- Emotional Health
- Tough Immune System
- Resilient Bodies
- Quick-Healing Injuries
- Healthy Hearing and Eye Sight

Hydration:

Kids are busy little people – always on the go – so it is important that they stay hydrated. Unfortunately, most kids don't drink nearly as much water as they should. Sure, they may take a few sips throughout the day, and if they are anything like my own kids, they probably ask for a glass of water 30 or so times at bedtime. But even then, moderate slurps are all they take in for the most part. Kids need hydration to help them stay energized, to help them concentrate, and most importantly, to keep their little bodies healthy. The hydrating value is yet another reason why a juicing regimen is excellent for kids. Not only are most juicing recipes made using water as one of the ingredients – but fresh fruits and vegetables are bursting with water!

Disease Prevention:

So much research has gone into how well juicing can prevent different diseases and illnesses. There have been thousands of studies done over the years, and many of these studies have concluded that juicing is beneficial in preventing and curing disease. Juicing has also shown to be beneficial in alleviating the symptoms of many ailments. Different fruits and vegetables offer different benefits, for instance – avocados can help reduce the symptoms associated with growing pains; spinach can help with earaches/ear infections; oranges can alleviate the symptoms of asthma as well as reduce the onset of attacks. The list goes on and on. We will look at the complete list of benefits a bit later in the book.

Helps Kids Develop Healthy Habits:

Research proves that adolescents who drink any amount of juice daily, made from fresh fruits and vegetables, have much lower consumptions of overall total dietary and saturated fats and higher consumptions of key nutrients, including B vitamins, vitamin C, Iron, potassium, fiber, and folate than those adolescents who do not drink any type of juice on a daily basis. Additionally, studies show that those children, ages 1 to 17, who drank at least 6-ounces of juice daily, also ate more whole fruit and vegetables and consumed fewer added sugars and fats.

There are many more reasons why juicing can benefit your child, and the items listed above are some of the most important benefits derived from juicing. Juicing can offer your child a lifetime of excellent health and overall well-being.

Sugar... Sugar... Everywhere!

Let's face it. With all the soda, candy, cupcakes, and brownies that surround our children, it can be hard to steer them towards healthier choices.

We know *why* our children should not consume large amounts of junk food, but in the minds of our children, junk food is fun food - and for a child, fun is everything.

I'm sure all of us have seen the look on our kids' faces whenever we encourage them to reach for the carrot sticks instead of the cookies. Mine look at me as though I've just punched Santa Claus square in the nose. Carrots aren't fun, Mom!

However, even though teaching our kids to appreciate fruits and veggies may be a battle at times, it is a battle worth fighting!

It can be tough to tell your kids no, especially when they look up to you with big bright eyes and pouty little mouths and ask oh so sweetly for sweets. It can be nearly impossible to turn them down, but at times, it is a necessary rejection.

On the other hand, it is vitally important to teach your children that sweets *can* be eaten in moderation. Some parents think that the best thing that they can do for themselves and their children is to not allow sweets or soda in the house, or to lock all the junk food in a cabinet. While this may work for a while, it does nothing to teach your children the skills of self-control and moderation. Also, avoiding junk food altogether can easily backfire when your child becomes an adult. Not having access to sweets during childhood may lead to a sugar addiction in adulthood. Think about it – your children are now 21 and living on their own. You never allowed them to have junk food as a child. Now as an adult, they realize they can eat whatever they want. So they begin stock piling candy, soda, ice cream, and cookies. They begin eating and eating and eating. We can *hope* that their newly found "adult-sized" common sense would eventually chime in and tell them "*that's enough,*" but it is possible that they could continue to eat it, and eat it, and eat it. If they had only been allowed to learn how to eat junk food in moderation as children, then those same learned habits might have followed them into adulthood – preventing the obsession to hoard and over-consume junk food.

Pediatricians, nutritionists, and scientists alike encourage allowing children to eat junk food in moderation. They claim that, in small amounts only, it is **not** harmful and that not allowing your children to eat junk food at all actually poses more short- and long-term risks than allowing sweets in moderation.

Many parents ask: *what is considered moderation for a child?* Well, it can vary depending on the child's age and activity level, but the general rule of thumb is to reduce junk food serving sizes to no more than the size of your child's palm. For a small child this might be 2 or 3 pieces of candy; for a teenager this might be 7 or 8 pieces of candy. How often they receive sweet treats is up to you, but you should not exceed more than one treat per day. Ideally, you should limit kids to no more than 3 to 4 sweets per week. This includes soda!

Teaching your children to only eat junk food in moderation also helps to instill self-control in your child, which will serve them greatly in many instances throughout their lives. Let your children choose the treat they would like to have, teach them about serving sizes and eventually, ease your kids into learning how to prepare their own servings in the size that is appropriate for their individual ages and bodies - with supervision, of course, as kids may be tempted to sneak in a little extra!

Juicing: Perfect Way to Kick the Soda Habit

Another important solution that juicing offers is that it is the perfect way to steer your kids away from soda and other dangerously sugary drinks. This includes many fruit juices that are available in stores today.

Be cautious when offering your children boxes, packets, or cups of fruit juices you find on the shelves in most stores. Even if they are labeled "real fruit juice", the truth is that they probably hold no more than 8-10% real fruit. Instead, they are filled with artificial flavorings, additives, tons of sugar, emulsifiers, colorings, food stabilizers, and other chemicals you do not want to put in your child's body.

On the other hand, with juicing, you know *exactly* what is going into your child. Most of the fruit juices that line the shelves in grocery stores are LOADED with sugar – lots and lots of it! Parents - don't be fooled! Many people think that if they just avoid buying beverages containing high fructose corn syrup then they are in the clear.

While it's true that all fruit juices that are labeled "100% fruit juice" do not always contain high fructose corn syrup, this doesn't necessarily mean that they are healthy for your child. Many of these juices contain a lot of sugar or artificial flavoring – neither of which are great for kids.

A while back, I was looking at the nutrition labels on some of the juices available in our local supermarket. One serving of store-brand grape juice, equal to 8 fl. ounces, had 42 grams of sugar! That's more sugar than there is in most 12 fl. oz cans of soda, which contains only 38 grams!

Say you think about handing your three year-old a Sippy cup full of store bought grape juice. You just as well might have filled the cup with a can of soda, and there would have been less sugar that way! Scary, isn't it?

I was also looking at bottles of apple juice, and I found one label that read "100% Apple Juice – No Sugar ADDED". Yet, for every eight fluid ounces of juice, there were already 28 grams of sugar! Can you imagine how much sugar would be in the juice had they added extra sugar?

Parents can be easily tricked with labels like this, so be very careful if you ever shop for store-bought fruit juices. Don't take the label at face value – investigate what the label says by looking at the nutrition label on the back of the juice. Compare that nutrition label with surrounding labels of the same type of juice to compare the nutrition data. Remember, just because a beverage is without high fructose corn syrup doesn't mean it's good for your kids.

You want to give your kids the best – so let's now compare nutrition labels of an 8 fl. oz. glass of store-bought 100% grape juice with the nutrition content of a 8 fl. oz. glass of raw juice:

100% Store-Bought Grape Juice	
Serving Size:	8 fl. oz.
Calories:	140
Total Fat:	0
Sodium:	15mg
Total Carbs:	38g
Sugar:	36g
Protein:	1g

Raw Juice with Concord Grapes and Wheatgrass	
Serving Size:	8 fl. oz.
Calories:	68
Total Fat:	0
Sodium:	2mg
Total Carbs:	14g
Sugar:	11g
Protein:	3.9g

The difference is quite amazing, considering how great the raw juice actually rates in taste comparison. I have done this particular recipe taste test with dozens of people over the years, adults and kids alike. For the test, I pour half a glass of store-bought 100% grape juice and a half a glass of the raw grape juice with wheatgrass. Neither glass is labeled. The participant tastes each juice and chooses the juice they think tastes the best. I cannot begin to describe how excited people get when they discover that they actually picked the raw juice – even over store-bought! I use store-bought grape juice a lot, mainly because it's a type of juice that *most* people like, especially kids. Many people think that maintaining a raw juicing regimen means that several times per day they have to choke back a nasty-tasting juice because it's good for them. They view juicing in the same way they would view having to take an awful-tasting medication. They think that something so healthy cannot possibly taste good. That's why they get so excited when they find out that they have actually chosen the raw juice.

People get excited and motivated about their juicing regimen, because they can now view drinking the juice as a treat, not a chore.

The Problem with Junk Food

Junk food is popular among people of all ages for obvious reasons. Not only does it taste great, but it is also very easy and convenient to prepare and eat –there's not much preparation that goes into opening up a bag of chips or a box of donuts. It's much easier to rely on a fast food drive-thru for dinner than it is to go home after a long day of work to prepare a healthy meal.

This is understandable, of course. We're all busy people. Many times we are tempted to take the easy road for meals and snacks. The convenience, along with the taste, can make junk food into an addiction – one that we can easily pass on to our children.

Junk food can lead to all sorts of health problems. It's very important to understand how an overdose of sugar, MSG, and artificial additives affects a child's body. Eating large amounts of junk food as a child paves the way to multiple health problems in later years.

Parents have heard all this before - more times that we can count. But I can't stress enough how important this information is.

Most junk food is loaded with sugar and fats. This makes them high in calories, and high calorie foods are usually low in nutritional value. When you eat junk food, you are basically filling your body with empty carbs, sugars, fats, and calories. This can lead to many health issues, particularly when the bulk of your diet is composed of fast food.

Some of the most common health risks associated with high junk food diets are:

> ➢ Weight gain
> ➢ Heart disease
> ➢ Heart attacks
> ➢ Strokes
> ➢ High cholesterol
> ➢ Clogged arteries
> ➢ Diabetes
> ➢ Kidney problems
> ➢ Liver damage
> ➢ Lack of energy and concentration
> ➢ Sugar and caffeine addiction

This is why giving junk food to your children only in moderation is so important. They are allowed to still have appropriate amounts of sweets, but the bulk of their diets are filled with nutritious foods. This counteracts the effects of any junk foods they may eat, resulting in fewer health risks.

It's okay to let your child eat that cupcake, just make sure they eat healthy throughout the rest of the day. Junk food is not bad in moderation; nor is it the enemy – as long as you control how much your child takes in!

There are different categories of junk food. Some junk food is healthier than others. For example, a bowl of gelatin topped with whipped cream is much healthier than deep fried donuts. It is possible to limit your child consumption of junk food to healthier versions of sweets.

Tips on Limiting Junk Food Intake

It can be very hard to keep your kids on the straight and narrow when it comes to eating healthy, especially when practically every commercial they watch on TV are tempting them to try some new type of junk food. There is a peculiar affinity that links junk food and children – it is our jobs as parents to teach kids to make healthy choices, to limit their intake of junk food, and to make sure that their relationship with junk food does not become habitual. We want our kids to view junk food as an occasional treat and *not* a daily occurrence. As parents, it is our duty to lead by example and not only limit our own intake of junk food, but to also monitor how much of it our children are consuming. There are several ways to make sure this happens.

Limit How Much Junk Food is Purchased:

If your typical grocery cart holds 75% junk food and 25% healthy choices, then you're buying way too much junk food. I always pay attention to the orders on the belt in the grocery store checkout line. It is almost laughable when I see a person purchasing sugary cereals, candy and cookies, potato chips, nutrient-sparse frozen entrees, and so on - but then, there in the midst of the junk food overhaul lies a single package of organic tofu. Now while I applaud the purchase of the tofu – balance is greatly needed. A package of cookies, a carton of ice cream, frozen pizzas and so on should only be purchased every once in a while as **a treat only** and as parents, you should mold your children's minds to view these items as just that... treats. A child should not view junk food as every day food – and it starts with you mom and dad! Just as we look around to view what other people are buying at the grocery store, our kids just may be taking notes as to what's in our own shopping cart – so lead by example!

It's also a good idea to do your grocery shopping when the kids are at school or when you are by yourself. A recent poll showed that moms tend to buy more junk food when their kids are shopping with them than they do when their shopping solo. Also, I know you've heard this before, but it is a rule that should ALWAYS be applied to your grocery shopping routine: **NEVER GO GROCERY SHOPPING ON AN EMPTY STOMACH!!!** When you shop while hungry, you are bound to purchase more sweets and junk food than you would if you were shopping on a recently fed tummy. When you are hungry – EVERYTHING looks good!

Meal Plans, Meal Plans, Meal Plans!

A great way to avoid consuming too much junk food is to make weekly or monthly meal plans and to stick to them! How many times have you gone into the grocery store without a list or plan and ended up walking out with a ton of stuff, except for the items you came for? You enter the store, knowing somewhat about what you need to buy, but nothing is set in stone. You hit the aisles – and think about what would be good for the week's meals. Because you don't have a shopping list, you wing it and end up usually with a bunch of stuff you don't need or you end up with too much junk food!

With a meal plan – you hit that store with an action plan. You know what you need and how much you need of it – you stay focused and on course and the chance of you being sidelined or distracted by the beckoning of junk food decreases immensely. When you go grocery shopping with a meal plan in hand – not only can you knock out a week or months' worth of groceries in that one visit – meal plans help you stick with a healthy diet for your family. You know what you are going to prepare each night and you have all the ingredients needed to prepare the night's meal – which will help reduce tons of stress and it will keep you from speed-dialing a pizza place at the last minute to order a pizza, because it's dinnertime and you don't have a clue as to what to make and your kids are acting as if the world is going to end if they don't get food in their bellies that very second. Take ten minutes once per week to create a meal plan – you will never again find yourself stressed out and winging it at the supermarket or in the kitchen!

Pack Healthy Snacks

Kids become hungry at the most inopportune times (standing in line at the bank, at the doctor's office, etc.,) which is why it is so important to always have healthy snacks ready to go at a moment's notice. Raisins, apple slices, rice cakes, grapes, granola, pretzels are all simple and mess-free ideas that will keep your kids happy and patient and will keep you from having to purchase snacks while out.

Prepare "Healthier" Versions of Junk Food Kids Love

Take a moment and think about your child's most favorite junk food. Is it bubblegum-flavored ice cream? Chocolate chip cookies? Corn dogs? Now take that food and do an internet search for healthier versions of that food. If your child's favorite snack is a type of processed snack cakes, then search for **"Healthier version of snack cake recipes."** Chances are a bunch of recipe options will pop up. I have made many healthy versions of my children's favorite junk food treats, and 9 times out of 10, they can't tell the difference! You will be amazed at all of the recipes you will find. They may take more time and energy to prepare for your kids then opening up a package of chocolate crème cookies, but the kiddies are worth it!

Now, again, even these healthier recipes should still be viewed as the "occasional treat." Just because they are healthier versions, doesn't make them healthy enough to eat every day. However, you will feel better about handing them over to your child when it's time for a treat.

Don't Take Your Children Off Junk Food Cold Turkey!

For those parents, whose children who eat junk food all the time or at least more often than they should – it's never too late to get your kids on a healthier nutritional path! However, the WORST thing you can do is cut out the junk food altogether immediately. Your kids are used to a particular diet, and making drastic changes too quickly will only make your children, and you, miserable.

Begin by cutting down the amount of junk food your child eats bit by bit each day and replacing the junk food with healthier snacks and meals. Make the elimination of junk food a gradual change, so slow that the kids barely notice. Replace or eliminate the junk food until you are down to no more than one small serving of junk food per day. From there, work your way down to one small serving 5 days per week, then 4 days, then every other day, until you reach your goal of one small serving of junk food no more than a few servings per week.

Slowly reducing your child's intake of junk food should prevent any major sugar crashes or temper tantrums. If your kids catch on and ask why they can't have as much junk food, explain it to them – tell them that some foods help your to grow taller and stronger, healthier and smarter, while some foods do not. Explain to them how important it is to eat the foods that will help them grow! Be sure to reassure them that the junk food is not going away completely – let them know that they can still eat the foods they like, just not as much or as often.

Never Use Junk Food as a Reward or Punishment

Many parents feel that straight A's on a report card means cupcakes or that a good soccer practice means a kid's meal at a fast food place. Or other parents may use junk food as a form of punishment – "You didn't do your chores, so NO ice cream!" You do not want to instill this thought process in your children. They will continue to think this way well into adulthood, where it could really hurt them, and potentially lead to weight issues and emotional struggles. They get a promotion at work – so the first thing they do is buy a big slice of cheesecake. Now that they're adults, there's nobody around to tell them otherwise. If ten great things happen in one week – then that's ten slices of cheesecake. Even worse, what if they are having a hard week? Things aren't going well. Maybe they made a big mistake at work or maybe they failed a test in college; maybe they got pulled over by the police and received an expensive ticket. When they did something wrong as kids, junk food was used as a reward. Now as adults they may use junk food in other ways, such as to self-medicate their sorrows.

Many adults are emotional eaters. It's important to teach your children from an early age that food should never be used as a reward or punishment – so that when they are adults, they will reward and "punish" themselves with healthier alternatives to junk food. Maybe a hard workout at the gym or a new haircut.

Praise and Celebrate Healthy Choices

Praise your children and celebrate with them any healthy choices they make when it comes to food - just don't celebrate with a cake! Make sure your children understand why the healthy food choice they made is so great and why it should be celebrated. Praise and celebration of good choices will motivate your children to make even more healthy choices in the future.

There you have it – you now know *why* juicing is great for kids, so now let's get into the specifics of the juicing and whole foods lifestyle. In the next few chapters, you will begin to learn and understand more about your children's nutritional needs and how to meet and exceed those needs with a juicing/whole foods lifestyle.

• • •

Keep in mind: While many adults can live on raw juice alone, kids need to supplement a whole foods diet with their juicing regimen to meet the needs of their growing bodies and developing minds. In Chapter 2, we will cover what a whole foods diet consists of and how to make it kid-friendly.

CHAPTER 2: A WHOLE FOODS DIET

What is a Whole Foods Diet?

A whole foods diet is comprised of foods that are as close to their natural form as possible – unprocessed, unrefined foods. An example of whole foods vs. non-whole foods would be brown rice vs. white rice. Since white rice is stripped of its germ, it is no longer natural – it has been refined, and along with being refined, the white rice has lost most of its nutritional value, including a majority of its fiber and various phytochemicals. **Phytochemicals** are chemicals naturally found in whole foods and they contain many protective and disease-fighting/preventative properties. When foods are processed they lose most of the phytochemicals they once possessed. Brown rice, however, maintains the whole kernel of the germ which means it retains its nutritious value.

In the beginning of time the only diet eaten by humans was a whole foods diet. As time progressed and we modernized, foods that were once natural and nutrient-rich began being processed and refined. When these foods began to be processed, they lost all that was good about them – fiber, vitamins, etc, and found additives that made them unhealthy – added sugars, trans fats and other fats, salt, and preservatives. Nowadays, the typical American diet is one comprised of mainly processed foods sprinkled here and there with some whole foods.

A whole foods lifestyle is one rich in foods such as:

- ✓ Whole Grains
- ✓ Vegetables
- ✓ Fruits
- ✓ Meats and Seafood (beef, chicken, fish, etc.)
- ✓ Legumes (beans, soybeans, peas, lentils, etc.)
- ✓ Nuts and Seeds
- ✓ Dairy (milk, yogurt, cheese, etc.)
- ✓ Eggs

A child needs these types of whole foods in order to be healthy and develop properly. As parents, we want to provide our kids with the best possible chance in life and teach them from an early age to be mindful of what they eat. This will help keep them strong and focused as they begin to leap hurdles and take on the world!

Whole Foods vs. Non Whole Foods

I want to reiterate that switching to a whole foods lifestyle does not necessarily mean that you will be taking away all of your children's favorite foods. There are so many ways you can give your kids many of their favorite foods using healthier whole foods versions. Many times your kids won't even know there is a difference. In all actuality, you might find that your kids prefer the whole foods version of their favorites. This is because whole foods taste so much better than processed foods – they are fresh and natural! They haven't been sealed away in a can or locked away in a freezer or injected with chemicals or placed on a shelf for who knows how long. Whole foods are the best of the best and, after all, your kids do deserve the best!

Take a look at the following list to get an idea of some examples of whole foods vs. foods that are not considered whole foods, but are childhood favorites. You will see that you can find close comparisons to just about every type of food that will help keep your kids smiling healthy smiles:

If Your Kids Want...	Offer Them This Instead...
Chicken Strips	Organic Grilled Chicken Breast Strips
Potato Chips	Popcorn
Milkshake	Fresh Fruit Smoothie
Macaroni and Cheese	Macaroni and Cheese (Just use whole grain macaroni noodles and natural cheeses)
Pizza	Pizza (Use whole grain dough, natural cheeses, quality meats, and fresh veggies.)
Cookies and Cream ice cream	Coconut milk ice cream topped with granola and chocolate chips
Corn cereal puffs cereal	Grab the whole grains version!
Anything else...	If there is not a whole grains version ready to buy, then Google the whole foods recipe or alternative to said food. Get creative!

How to Begin a Whole Foods Lifestyle

Many parents want to help their kids eat healthier, they are just at a loss over where or how to begin. There is one rule you should follow when beginning a whole foods lifestyle:

Keep it simple!

Use the following tips to get started:

Step One: Start out by buying whole foods at the grocery store. Remember: whole foods are foods that are as close to their natural state as possible. This means food that have not been processed or refined. These are foods without added sugar, preservatives, additives, artificial flavorings, and so on. Select fresh fruits and vegetables, natural dairy products (for those whose kids crave chocolate milk – there is organic chocolate milk available), whole grains, and so on. Try to avoid refined white rice and pastas, packaged meals and snacks, sugary cereals, enriched white breads, and other processed choices.

Step Two: Look for free-range and hormone-free versions of meats, eggs, and other animal products. You may have to purchase your meats from a store such as Whole Foods Market or Sprouts, or go to the local butcher. Many grocery stores only offer meats that have been treated with antibiotics or other substances, or from animals that were fed a nutrient-deficient diet. There are some supermarkets that are changing to free-range, hormone-free meat products – call ahead to see if your preferred grocer offers these higher-quality meats.

Step Three: Don't be too consumed by what's on the food label – this can become confusing, so when starting out, just focus on choosing foods which are fresh and natural. As you become more familiar with whole foods vs. non whole foods, you can begin to "shop" the labels. There are so many whole foods cook books and online recipes and meal plans that can make preparing a whole foods menu a snap for your family. Search online for whole foods dishes you believe your family would love and go crazy experimenting with different whole foods dishes. Most dishes can be prepared in less than 30 minutes, so don't fear that feeding your family a healthy diet means you will never again leave the kitchen, this isn't so. You be delighted when you see the smiling, approving faces of your family when they ask for seconds! By the way – there are many recipes for delicious whole foods desserts!

Step Four: Don't confuse a whole foods diet with a raw foods diet – the two are very different. You can absolutely cook or bake every meal! You do not have to eat anything raw if you do not want to. When experimenting with whole foods dishes, try adding in spices and natural flavors. Have fun with cooking and baking whole foods. Eventually you will find yourself creating your own signature whole foods dish! It is absolutely recommended that you combine fruits and vegetables, meats, eggs, whole grains, and dairy together in soups, casseroles, stir fry, stews, salads, and other dishes.

Guidelines to Maintaining a Whole Foods Diet

Here are some helpful guidelines that will help you in providing your little ones with the type of diet that will keep them growing like weeds!

Always Opt for Whole Grains: There are whole grain versions of just about everything nowadays. If your kids refuse to eat anything but white bread, choose the "whole grain white". This version of bread looks like white bread, but it is whole grain bread in disguise. This is one way to win the white bread battle while keeping your kids happy! Whole grain pastas are another great choice – when making spaghetti (a childhood favorite) use whole grain spaghetti; your kids will be none the wiser. Choose brown rice over white rice. Use whole grain oats, millet, and quinoa in stir fries, cookies, and baked goods. Whenever possible, replace refined grains with whole grains. Processed grains, such as white flour, have drastic consequences on a child's health, such as a rise in insulin and blood sugar levels in children, which could easily lead to diabetes and childhood obesity.

Pick Out High Quality Proteins: Protein is an essential part of our children's diets. Protein acts as a fuel source to help keep our kids going strong at school and at play. Additionally, the rate at which kids grow and physical activity levels will increase the amount of protein that their bodies need. The more active the kid, the more protein is needed. Protein also helps the body heal faster from injury or after any trauma, such as post-surgery. Protein is right up there with the most important nutrients our children require as they grow.

People who are protein deficient are at increased risk for severe malnutrition and mental illnesses, as well as a disorder referred to as Kwashiorkor. Kwashiorkor is more common in areas of famine and poor food supply such as in developing countries where severe malnutrition is an epidemic, and is not as common among American children. However, there have been nearly 300 cases in America since 2002 and this disorder can affect any child that is severely protein deficient.

Symptoms of Kwashiorkor include severe diarrhea, failure to thrive in children, low-activity or inactivity, flaky skin and edema of the legs and belly, apathy, fatty liver, and more. It is a tragic disorder which devastates the lives of children. Additionally, children do not necessarily need to be from low-income areas to be affected by Kwashiorkor. There have been several cases where children from affluent communities have also been affected by this disorder. Children with chronic diseases and children who are frequently hospitalized for prolonged periods of time are also at a higher risk for contracting this disorder. Some disorders which increase a child's risk of being affected by Kwashiorkor include cystic fibrosis, cardiovascular disease, end stage renal failure, any types of cancer/leukemia, genetic disorder/disease, and neurological disease. Children who are sick but remain undiagnosed, or children with multiple diagnoses, are also at risk for the disorder. Once a sick child is affected with Kwashiorkor, their chances of a speedy and full recovery diminishes greatly.

Different types of protein can be found in meats and seafood, nuts and seeds, tofu, eggs, and beans. Be sure to pick protein sources that are organic and hormone free. Look for labels that say things like "grass fed beef" or choose omega-3 eggs.

Choose a rainbow of fruits and veggies: When it comes to produce, each color holds special health benefits. Instead of only picking out green vegetables or yellow fruits, choose a variety of fruits and vegetables in an array of colors. Take a look at each table below for a quick glimpse at some of the many benefits each color holds:

RED			
Benefits:			
Full of antioxidants; Contains lycopene which offers a variety of health benefits including heart health, cancer preventative agents, memory health, etc.; Boosts immune function; Promotes strong and healthy skin, bones, and teeth			
Red Apples	Watermelon	Beets	Red Pepper
Tomatoes	Red Kidney Beans	Strawberries	Cranberries

Green			
Benefits:			
Speeds up metabolic rate; Rich in folate and lutein which aid in many things, including healthy vision; Aids in the treatment and prevention of many ailments and diseases; Darker green veggies offer a huge vitamin boost			
Green Apples	Kiwi Fruit	Avocados	Broccoli
Green Beans	Sweet Peas	Asparagus	Spinach

Yellow/Orange			
Benefits:			
High in Vitamin A, C, and Folate; Promotes strong immune system; Healthy eyes and vision; Improves memory and overall mental function.			
Apricots	Lemons	Cantaloupe	Oranges
Carrots	Pumpkin	Sweet Potatoes	Yellow Lentils

White/Brown/Tan			
Benefits:			
Rich in Potassium and Allicin; Promotes heart health; Helps alleviate childhood "growing pains"; Helps keep adolescents healthy throughout puberty.			
Coconut	Dates	Brown Pears	Cauliflower
Cauliflower	Kohlrabi	White Onions	Mushrooms

Purple/Black/Blue			
Benefits:			
Aids in healthy eyes and vision; Helps treat and prevent aches and pains; Promotes fast healing; Healthy growth and development			
Blueberries	Plums	Purple Grapes	Black Olives
Eggplant	Purple Asparagus	Black Beans	Blackberries

Always choose fresh foods over canned or frozen - Always avoid purchasing irradiated foods, foods with growth hormones, additives, and/or preservatives, or foods which have been genetically engineered in any way. Instead, buy organic foods or look for a label on the foods which reads "GMO Free".

Avoid hydrogenated oils or trans-fatty acids whenever possible- Hydrogenated oils and trans-fatty acids can be found in nearly every processed food. Buy oils such as extra virgin olive oil, coconut oil, grapeseed oil, and flax oil - be sure to avoid canola oil! They cost a little more, but the health benefits are well worth the price difference. Healthy oils help your body absorb the minerals found in foods.

Try sea vegetables - Sea veggies are nutritional powerhouses. They help the body rid itself of the daily toxins and harmful chemicals we come in contact with on a day to day basis. Try sea vegetables such as kelp, arame, nori, wakame, and dulse.

Making the Transition to Whole Foods

Many children have a diet based on processed foods, refined grains, and high amounts of sugar and fats. Taking a child from this type of diet to a whole foods diet can be trying at best, especially when dealing with the older the child. However, it is important to transition a child to a diet where the above foods are only consumed in moderation. A diet high in sugar, fats, and processed foods can lead to serious nutritional deficiencies. Balance out the occasional sweets with a balanced and nutritional whole foods diet.

There are also many little tips and tricks that you can use to make the transition easier for the kids. Brown rice, for example, is an excellent source of nutrition and it can be added to a variety of dishes. A great way to introduce brown rice to your kids is by first mixing it with white rice (half and half), your kids will see that the taste is not all that different and they will be more willing to eat brown rice solo the next time around.

In addition, there are many whole grain versions of your children's' favorite foods – cookies, crackers, etc. There are also many favorite cereals that are also now made with whole grains. Keep an eye out for these – they are a great way to give your children the foods they want while being able to maintain the whole foods diet. Just keep an eye on the nutrition label to make sure the sugar content is not too crazy.

What's most important is that you make the transition as stress-free and fun as possible, for both you and your kids. You do not want to make the change seem troublesome or difficult or too stressful – remember that your kids are always watching to see how you will react to something. For their sake, make the transition to whole foods seem like an adventure. Even if you are a little stressed out, confused, or not sure how to begin – fake it. Don't let the kiddos smell your fear! The next set of guidelines should help reduce some of the stress.

Guidelines for the Transition to a Whole Foods Diet

When changing a child's diet, it is important to take baby steps. Make the change gradual. This will not only prevent your child from noticing a dramatic change off the bat and throwing a fit, but it will also allow their bodies to adjust to the changes accordingly. You don't want their bodies to experience too much too fast, this could lead to tummy aches, constipation, or diarrhea, among other uncomfortable ailments. The best way to go about making the transition is to do the following:

Week One: Make one meal per day for the first week a whole foods meal – with absolutely NO processed foods or refined grains. Snacks and other meals continue as usual.

Week Two: Make breakfast and dinner a whole foods meal. If your children eat lunch at school, that's fine. If they take lunch to school – then keep the lunches to what your kids are typically used to. Snacks continue as usual.

Week Three: For week 3, try making all three meals whole food meals. Snacks continue as usual.

Week Four: This is it! Now it's time to make all three meals of the day whole foods meals AND it is also time to make the 2 to 3 snacks your child has per day whole foods snacks. There are many types of whole foods snacks your child can eat that they will love such as: string cheese, beef jerky, granola, granola bars, trail mix, nuts and seeds, yogurt parfaits, fresh fruit, apple slices (you can even add some caramel for dipping), and the list goes on and on.

Note: Once week four is in play, you can begin giving your kids sweets and processed foods in moderation. Allow them to choose junk food to eat no more than 1 to 3 times per week. In addition, those families who choose to eat five small meals per day as oppose to 3 larger meals, the same transition guidelines apply, just account for the amount of meals and snacks your children eat per day and begin substituting whole foods a meal or two at a time.

Whole Foods Lifestyle: The Sky's the Limit!

Once you become familiar with the whole foods lifestyle, you will never run out of ideas for the next meal or snack. It may seem at first that the grocery store is packed full of more processed foods than whole foods. You have just been used to buying from the areas stocked full of processed and refined foods. Remember: For a whole foods lifestyle - - the outer perimeter (along each wall) of the supermarket is your best friend. These are the areas that typically house the produce section, deli, meat counter, and so on. Try to avoid the inner aisles as much as possible! When you shop at health food stores such as Whole Foods Market or Sprouts, the sky's the limit – the entire layout of the store is dedicated to the whole foods lifestyle. So go on and explore all that's available for the whole foods family!

CHAPTER 3: YOUR CHILD'S NUTRITIONAL NEEDS

Know Your Child's Daily Nutritional Needs

Understanding your child's daily nutritional needs makes following a juicing and whole foods lifestyle much easier. Meeting your child's nutritional needs now can lead to a lifetime of good nutritional habits. Each child is different, and no one knows your child like you do. So while the nutritional requirements listed throughout this chapter are according to the American Pediatric Nutritional Database, each child is different and may have different nutritional requirements. Depending on how active your child is, their age and sex, allergies and ailments, their nutritional needs may vary. Therefore use the information listed in this chapter as a starting point only. Adjust the information appropriately to meet the needs of your own child.

Many parents over-think their child's daily nutritional needs. They think that if their child is short on one or more of their daily requirements, the whole house will come tumbling down. This not only stresses parents out, but it can put unneeded stress on children as well. When meeting your child's daily needs, don't worry about being exact. Don't worry about being perfect. Don't force your children to clean their plates – it's okay! All these nutritional requirements are in place for is for parents to use as a guide in making sure kids get the types of foods their bodies need to grow and develop. If your child doesn't finish his glass of milk at breakfast and it is really bothering you, then try adding a piece of string cheese or yogurt to one of his daily snacks to make up for it. Don't put stress on yourself and your child by forcing him to finish the milk – it's really not worth the wasted energy. Your child will be fine and that missing dairy need can be made up for later.

On the other hand, there are parents who do not worry about making sure their children's daily needs are met – this doesn't make them bad parents at all. In most cases, these parents feel as if their children's needs are already being met by the foods they currently eat and they don't feel as if they need to abide by any set of "requirements" or "standards." You might be surprised at how much better your child feels and behaves when she's met her daily nutrition requirements, though. There's no harm in giving it a try!

Whether you obsess over your children's nutritional needs or you aren't concerned with them at all – it is important to find a balance. Somewhere in between the two scenarios is where you want to be when it comes to meeting your children's nutritional needs.

The very basic requirements that you should be meeting for your children are:

- 3 meals per day.
- 2 nutritious snacks.
- Feed your child a variety of foods.
- Make sure there is a somewhat even balance between the amount of food your child eats and their level of physical activity.
- Feed your child a diet full of whole grains, vegetables, and fruit.
- Keep your child's diet low of added sugars, high salt contents, trans fat, saturated fat, and cholesterol (remember, your child's body needs fats to grow and develop properly – just try to fill them up with more good fats than bad fats).
- Make sure your child's diet has enough calcium and iron on a daily basis to meet the needs of their growing bodies. Whole milk is an excellent choice for growing children,

and can actually help to curb obesity and assist in weight management.

- Try to avoid as many processed foods, soda (and other forms of caffeine), sugary fruit juices, and other carbonated drinks, as possible.

As we covered earlier, a child's daily nutritional requirements varies based on different factors, including age, sex of child, and physical activity levels. For instance, your 16 year-old son's diet requirements are going to differ from your 6 year-old daughter's diet needs. Below are a set of guidelines to give you an idea of a child's nutritional needs based on their age.

Ages 2 to 3: Girls and Boys	
Calories	1,000 to 1,400 depending on growth/activity levels
Protein	2 to 4 ounces
Fruits	1 to 1½ cups
Vegetables	1 to 1½ cups
Grains	3 to 5 ounces
Dairy	2 to 2½ cups
Ages 4 to 8: Girls	
Calories	1,200 to 1,800 depending on growth/activity levels
Protein	3 to 5 ounces
Fruits	1 to 1½ cups
Vegetables	1½ to 2½ cups
Grains	4 to 6 ounces
Dairy	2½ to 3 cups
Ages 4 to 8: Boys	
Calories	1,200 to 2,000 depending on growth/activity levels
Protein	3 to 5½ ounces
Fruits	1 to 2 cups
Vegetables	1½ to 1½ cups
Grains	4 to 6 ounces
Dairy	2½ to 3 cups
Ages 9 to 13: Girls	
Calories	1,400 to 2,200 depending on growth/activity levels
Protein	4 to 6 ounces
Fruits	1½ to 2 cups

Vegetables	1½ to 3 cups
Grains	5 to 7 ounces
Dairy	2½ to 3 cups
Ages 9 to 13: Boys	
Calories	1,600 to 2,600 depending on growth/activity levels
Protein	5 to 6½ ounces
Fruits	1½ to 2 cups
Vegetables	2 to 3½ cups
Grains	5 to 9 ounces
Dairy	3 cups
Ages 14 to 18: Girls	
Calories	1,800 to 2,400 depending on growth/activity levels
Protein	5 to 6½ ounces
Fruits	1½ to 2 cups
Vegetables	2½ to 3 cups
Grains	6 to 8 ounces
Dairy	3 cups
Ages 14 to 18: Boys	
Calories	2,000 to 3,200 depending on growth/activity levels
Protein	5½ to 7 ounces
Fruits	2 to 2½ cups
Vegetables	2½ to 4 cups
Grains	6 to 10 ounces
Dairy	3 cups

Child-Sized Portions: Size DOES Matter!

An issue that many parents have is that they are uncertain of what child-sized portions actually are. I cannot believe it when I am at a restaurant and I see a 3 year-old with as much food on his plate as his dad! This is not okay! When you feed your child adult-sized portions, you are building poor habits that follow them into adulthood and eventually parenthood, when they themselves will be giving their own toddler a full-size Porterhouse!

Keep a close eye on HOW MUCH your child is eating at every meal. Don't worry, your children won't starve if you begin to cut down their portion sizes – they will actually thrive because of it. If you have a child who eats like there's no tomorrow and who seems to be never be filled up – there are things you can do. Try feeding them more mini meals throughout the day instead of three big meals. Another idea is to give them a full glass of water to drink before they begin eating. If neither of these tips help, try to remember, when kids go through growing spurts they tend to have bigger appetites. If after they finish their meal, they ask for seconds – give them a 8-ounce glass of water, have them drink it and if after about 5 to 10 minutes they are still hungry, even after drinking the water then give them seconds. This time around, cut their typical portion size in half. There is nothing wrong with giving your kids second helpings, just remember – it usually takes about 10 minutes for the food to settle in your stomach and your stomach to signal to your brain that you are full. So have your kids wait a few minutes to make sure they really are still hungry. The glass of water in between portions will help their food to settle faster which will help them feel fuller. Unmanaged portion sizes are one of the main causes of childhood obesity. It is exceedingly important to make sure your children are eating the appropriate amounts of food.

Keep in mind that the following guide is to be used as an example only. Your child's portion sizes may need to increase or decrease depending on her own daily requirements.

Meats/Seafood	3 ounces	Deck of Cards
Pasta/Rice	½ cup	Tennis Ball / Ice Cream Scoop
Bread	1 slice	CD Case
Peanut Butter	2 tablespoons	Ping-Pong Ball
Vegetables	½ cup	Light Bulb or Rounded Handful
Cheese	1 ounce	Four Dice
Dried Fruit	1 ounce	One Egg
Nuts	1 ounce	Ping-Pong Ball

A good rule-of-thumb: if you're not quite sure about a type of food is to **portion out the food according to the size of your child' palm.** This will get you nearly perfect to the correct portion size. When it comes to portioning out crackers, cookies, cereal, and almost every other type of processed/packaged food – look at the food label and find the serving size for that food. The portion size is per serving, this may be more or less than the portion size that is appropriate for your child as these are generalized portions and not according to sex and age of child. For instance, if a bag of chips has a serving size of 32 chips – then that may be a bit much for your 7 year-old – so break it down to a portion size more fitting for your child. It is important to just use your best judgment when divvying out these types of food portions.

The following food label is a sample from the Food and Drug Administration which makes it simple to see how to determine the serving size of a particular food. Remember when reading a food label that the information provided is PER SERVING.

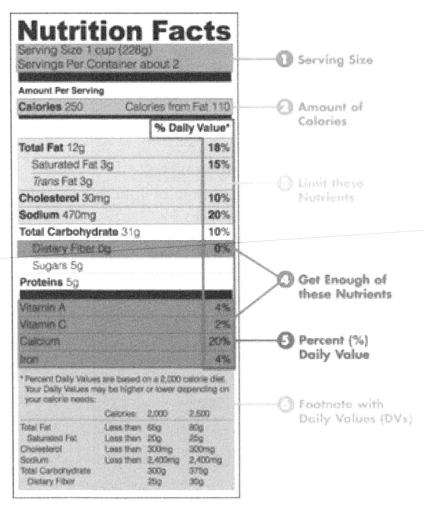

Nutrients Children Need to Thrive

Children need certain types of nutrients daily to help them grow and develop properly. Without these nutrients, not only might your child have issues in the vital areas of growth and development, but they also may have more health issues, both physical and psychological.

When you are at the point where you begin creating your own juicing recipes for your kids, or you begin experimenting with different types of produce and additives, be sure to pay attention to the types of nutrients being offered in the juices you are creating. Take a look at the following list of nutrients your child needs on a daily basis in order to reach their full potential.

Protein: Your children need protein daily. It not only gives them energy and helps with growth, coordination, and movement but it also helps kids develop healthy eyes and strong gums, it builds and develops strong muscles and glands. Protein also helps to create antibodies which can help a child's body fight off infection and disease.

Adding Protein to Raw Juice: To add protein to your child's juicing regimen (or when preparing green smoothies), use the following sources:

- Bananas
- Blackberries
- Blueberries
- Spinach

Adding Protein to Green Smoothies:
- Milk
- Yogurt
- Seeds and nuts
- A scoop of protein powder

Vitamin A: Vitamin A is important to kids for many reasons, healthy eyesight being one of them. Between 250,000 and 500,000 children worldwide go blind each year due to a lack of Vitamin A. Vitamin A deficiency leads to growth and development issues as well, and it can make the body unable to resist or fight off infection.

Adding Vitamin A to Raw Juice: To add Vitamin A to your child's juicing regimen (or when preparing green smoothies), use the following sources:

- Broccoli
- Cantaloupe
- Carrots
- Apricots
- Sweet Potatoes
- Winter Squash

Vitamin B6: Children (especially infants) need Vitamin B6 for a variety of reasons, such as brain development and a healthy immune system. A lack of Vitamin B6 can lead to hearing problems and seizures in young children and a plethora of other ailments in children of all ages.

Adding Vitamin B6 to Raw Juice: To add Vitamin B6 to your child's juicing regimen, use the following sources:

- Avocado
- Bananas
- Carrots
- Spinach
- Wheat Germ

Vitamin B12: Vitamin B12 does many things for the human body, including making DNA and keeping blood and nerve cells healthy. It also helps kids with their energy and endurance levels. Vitamin B12 is mostly found in meats and seafood, however, there are some other food sources rich in B12.

Adding Vitamin B12 to Raw Juice: To add Vitamin B12 to your child's juicing regimen, use the following sources:

- Spirulina
- Sea vegetables, such as seaweed
- A drop or two of liquid B12 in your child's juice

Adding Vitamin B12 to Green Smoothies:

- Milk or Soy Milk
- Yogurt
- Whey Protein Powder
- Sea vegetables, such as:
  - Atlantic Wakame
  - Dulse
  - Nori
  - Sea Lettuce

Vitamin C: All kids need Vitamin C. It not only keeps their immune system healthy, but it also does many other things to help your child's body growing and functioning properly. Remember: Your child's body cannot store Vitamin C; therefore you need to give your child Vitamin C on a daily basis so that your child's body has enough of it.

Adding Vitamin C to Raw Juice: To add Vitamin C to your child's juicing regimen (or when preparing green smoothies), use the following sources:

- All types of berries
- Cantaloupe
- Grapefruit
- Kiwi
- Leafy greens
- Lemons
- Oranges
- Papayas
- Strawberries
- Sweet red peppers
- Tomatoes

Calcium: Children need calcium for strong bones and healthy teeth and for many other reasons. Many parents think that the best source of calcium for their children is milk. While milk is an excellent source of calcium, it is not appropriate for your child's juicing regimen. There are many sources of calcium that you can use to make scrumptious raw juice and green smoothies.

Adding Calcium to Raw Juice: To add Calcium to your child's juicing regimen (or when preparing green smoothies), use the following sources:

- Green Leafy Vegetables, such as:
  - Kale
  - Spinach
  - Collard Greens
  - Turnip Greens

Adding Calcium to Green Smoothies:

- Dates
- Green leafy vegetables
- Milk

- Nuts and seeds
- Oranges
- Raisins
- Soybeans
- Yogurt

Folic Acid: This nutrient is a kid's requirement for a variety of reasons. Folic acid is needed for the production and division of healthy cells. Folic acid is vital in the production of blood cells, hair cells, skin cells, bone cells, and nerve cells.

Adding Folic Acid to Raw Juice: To add folic acid to your child's juicing regimen, use the following sources:

- Beets
- Green leafy vegetables
- Oranges
- Papayas
- Root vegetables
- Legumes

Iron: Iron is very important for kids, as it helps produce hemoglobin. Parents whose children are anemic or whose teenage girls are menstruating need to pay close attention to ensure they are getting enough iron in their diets daily. **Note:** Avoid feeding your child too many high-fiber cereals, as an overdose can prevent the absorption of iron.

Adding Iron to Raw Juice: To add iron to your child's juicing regimen, try using the following sources:

- All Fruits

- Basil
- Green leafy vegetables
- Parsley
- Prunes
- Pumpkin

Magnesium: Magnesium is vital for your child's general health and development. Magnesium also helps in keeping a child's bones, heart, nervous system, and muscles strong and properly functioning. Magnesium also aids in keeping immune systems healthy.

Adding Magnesium to Raw Juice: To add magnesium to your child's juicing regimen, try using the following sources:

- All Greens:
    - Spinach
    - Spirulina
    - Chlorella
- Banana
- Beet Greens
- Collard Greens
- Cucumber
- Grapefruit
- Papayas
- Pumpkin
- Rutabaga

- Squash
- Wheat Germ

Zinc: Kids need zinc for healthy skin, hair, and nails. Zinc also removes any excess carbon dioxide from your child's body.

Adding Zinc to Raw Juice: To add zinc to your child's juicing regimen, try using the following sources:

- Apricots
- Avocado
- Carrots
- Collard Greens
- Kale
- Prunes
- Spinach
- Summer Squash
- Swiss Chard

Essential Fatty Acids: Your child needs these fatty acids for proper growth and development, particularly neurological development and sensory system health and maturity.

Adding Essential Fatty Acids to Raw Juice: To add essential fatty acids to your child's juicing regimen, try using the following sources:

- Avocados
- Collard Greens

- Flaxseed Oil
- Kale
- Mustard Greens
- Spinach

All of the nutrients your child needs may seem a bit overwhelming starting out, but the easiest way to ensure your children's good health is to provide them with a variety of fruits and vegetables daily; in their juices, and on their plates. Fresh fruits and vegetables are the best sources of vitamins and minerals.

CHAPTER 4: JUICING BASICS

Juicing and Your Child

Ah-ha, finally! The moment we've been waiting for! It's time to learn the steps to take in order to get juicing for our little ones! It's just as important to learn how to get our little ones on board with juicing. Some kids adapt very well to juicing. Some kids – not so much – but don't fear! This book will help guide you through all of the battles you may face in getting your child on a steady juicing regimen. Throughout this chapter we will discuss:

- Basic guide on juicing for kids
- Safe juicing methods for children
- How much juice each day is safe for your kids
- How to get fussy or picky kids on a juicing regimen
- Much, much more!

Basics to Juicing for Kids

The first, and really, only major rule when it comes to juicing for kids is to:

Account for their Age.

A child's tummy is much more sensitive than an adult's stomach. This is especially true when introducing kids to new types of food. Children ages 3 and up should be able to safely consume raw fruit and vegetable juices with little issues. Children under 2 years of age, particularly those that are breastfed, do not need to be on a juicing regimen. This is due to several reasons. The first being that when a child is born their little bodies are nutritional powerhouses and through breastfeeding and baby foods, they remain nutrition-packed little people until they reach the age when they begin to be introduced to processed foods and worldly toxins. This is typically around 3 years of age. Therefore, parents of children under two – it is recommended that you hold off until age three. However, it is okay to give a child who is at least 12 months old little sips of fresh juice here and there. That way, when they hit a full juicing regimen, their little bodies will have already been introduced to the juices.

Juicing fresh fruits and vegetables is something you can do for your children which can hold benefits that will last their entire lifetime. Don't worry about adding some form of fruit to every juice you make in order to sweeten the taste for your child. Some parents worry that this could lead to childhood obesity. This couldn't be farther from the truth. Fresh fruits contain natural sugars which are very simple for your child's body to assimilate. So go on and mix in those fresh fruits, if that makes your child more willing to drink it!

Here are some more guidelines to keep in mind before you begin juicing:

- Give your children a full glass of raw fruit juice in the morning. This will give them the carbs needed to fuel their day. In the afternoon, switch to partial raw green juice (vegetables/greens mixed with fruit to sweeten) or full raw green juice (vegetables/greens only). Avoid full fruit juice in the late afternoon or evening as this can give your child a surge of energy right before bed, making it difficult for them to sleep.

- During the first 2 weeks of a juicing regimen, for children ages 12 and under, dilute each juice with a little water. For instance, dilute a 6-ounce juice with a ¼ cup of water;

an 8-ounce juice with 1/3 cup of water; a 10-ounce juice with ½ cup of water; a 12-ounce juice with ¾ cup of water. This will help to keep any adverse reactions due to the changes in their diet to a minimum.

- You may find that your children end up preferring raw juice over any other drinks. However, for the health and well-being of your child, raw juices should only be consumed in moderation. Be sure to keep your kids drinking plenty of water to keep from becoming dehydrated.

- Even though fresh fruit juices contain natural sugars, your children are still at risk for cavities and tooth decay so it is important to follow up each juice with a small glass of water to help flush out any sugars left behind in their mouths.

- The best time to give your child their juice when first starting out is first thing in the morning with their breakfast. The juices may create a fluctuation in your child's levels of energy, which is more noticeable in the beginning. If you combine their juice with breakfast, the food will help to slow the absorption of the juice in your child's body which in turn will help to steady out their energy levels. Furthermore, you should never give your child a juice close to meal times. Juices are very filling; so much so that consuming one close to mealtime may prevent your child from eating their food. This can deprive their bodies of the nutrients the food would have provided.

- For the first 7 to 10 days of your child's juicing regimen, it is important to monitor your child closely. Look for any changes in health or behavior. Listen for complaints of upset tummies, constipation, or diarrhea. Look for any reactions to certain types of fruits or vegetables. For example, say you notice that every time you put mango in your child's juice that they have an upset tummy. Either adjust the amount of mango used or use mango only as a sweetener in raw vegetable juices.

Juice Poisoning

Many children are allergic to different types of foods. It can be difficult as parents to determine if our children have any allergies to foods. Young children are most at risk for reacting to a food allergy mainly because they are being introduced to new foods all the time. Unfortunately, most of the time, the only way to know if your child has a food allergy is once they have had an allergic reaction to a food.

When it comes to fresh fruits and vegetables, most children consume them safely without any issues. However, some fruits and vegetables are so high in antioxidants that they could cause a reaction in some children. When giving your child green juice (juices solely made from greens) it is important to go slow and in very small amounts. Greens are a potent detoxifier and packed with nutrition – if introduced too fast, your child could easily feel ill after consuming the green juice and their bodies will begin to absorb and detoxify the greens at a much faster rate than other types of juice. In the recipe section of this book, you will find some simple green juice recipes that will not wreak havoc on your child's body. If offering your children fruits or vegetables for the first time (especially if your child has a history of food allergies to various foods) always test the produce by cutting them a small piece to eat. **Wait 15 to 30 minutes for any signs of allergic reaction.** Once you determine that no reaction occurs, you can safely begin adding these fruits and vegetables to your child's juicing regimen:

- Kiwis
- Papayas
- Peaches
- Cherries

- Citrus Fruit
- Pineapple
- Strawberries
- Tomatoes
- Wheatgrass

Symptoms of Juice Poisoning

When offering your child new types of fruits and vegetables for the first time, particularly those fruits and vegetables from the list above, always monitor your children for signs of allergic reaction. The following are some of the common symptoms associated with juice poisoning that you need to watch out for:

- Swelling tongue and/or lips
- Bluish tint to skin (means that your child is not getting enough oxygen)
- Sneezing
- Stuffy or runny nose
- Cough
- Shortness of breath
- Itchy and/or splotchy skin

Difference Between Food Allergy and Food Intolerance

It is very important to know the difference in your child being **ALLERGIC** and them being **INTOLERANT** of a particular food. Being ALLERGIC to food can be life threatening and often involves some very serious symptoms, from swelling of the tongue to trouble breathing. The onset of symptoms to food allergies are almost immediate (typically within 5 to 15 minutes time). Being INTOLERANT of food, while the symptoms are uncomfortable, they can often be treated easily at home with very minimal intervention. The onset of symptoms for food intolerance are often delayed (often not appearing for hours, sometimes even days later). Symptoms of FOOD INTOLERANCE include:

- Tummy Aches
- Constipation
- Flatulence (Gas)
- Bloating
- Colic

In more serious cases, food intolerance can even bring about:

- Vomiting
- Diarrhea

You need to look out for those kids who are chronic picky eaters. Sometimes food intolerance come across in the form of picky eating. Kids who are picky eaters may not tell you about any symptoms they are having; they just refuse to eat certain foods because it hurts their tummies or causes them other discomfort. If your children have been picky eaters most of their lives, there may be more to it. Next time they refuse to eat a certain food, investigate – but don't interrogate! Calmly ask them why they do not like the food. Try to gently determine if they won't eat the food because they are intolerant of it. Children with a history of intolerance to certain foods may have a build-up of bacteria in their digestive tract which can easily lead to symptoms of intolerance. Ask your pediatrician about putting your child on a combination of Vitamin C and probiotics to reverse your child's intolerance to certain types of foods.

Tips to Minimize the Occurrence of Juice Poisoning

When preparing your child's juicing regimen, take the following steps to avoid the risk of juice poisoning:

> ➤ Choose organic fruits and vegetables as often as you are able. Organic produce is more expensive, however, you can be certain when giving your children organic produce that the produce is safe and free of chemicals or pesticides. Another option is to purchase a gear juicer. The gear juicer will allow you to continue buying regular produce as the juicer can separate the most, if not all, of the pesticides and other chemicals from the juices.

> ➤ Use fruits and vegetables that are just at the right degree of ripeness. When you offer your children food that is unripe, almost ripe, or overripe, you run the risk of juice poisoning. Produce products are more allergenic if they are not properly ripe, thus increasing your child's risk of a reaction. If you are unsure if a certain type of produce is ripe, ask the produce clerk at the grocery store or search online how to tell if produce is ripe. Note: The part of a fruit or vegetable that is most allergenic is the skin. For children with a history of food allergies, it might be wise to peel or cut the skin off of produce before juicing it.

> ➤ Make sure that you properly wash produce that is non-organic. Taking the following steps will ensure that the produce is washed thoroughly:

>> 1. Place 2 tablespoons of Apple Cider Vinegar and 1 teaspoon of salt into a sink of cool water.

>> 2. Soak the produce in the water for 15 minutes.

3. After about 15 minutes, the water should smell fairly awful. This is the result of the chemicals and pesticides having been removed.

4. Finally, rinse the produce off well with cool water. Prepare the produce for juicing.

➢ Your juicer must be cleaned very well between each use. Never store it away until it is completely dry as this could result in the growth and spread of bacteria.

Juicing Regimen for Picky Eaters

Getting kids to eat right in general can be tough, but getting picky eaters to eat right can be seemingly impossible. So many parents feel helpless when they have kids who are picky eaters. They are so concerned that their child eat something, anything, that they often give in to junk foods so that their kids are at least putting *something* into their mouths. The problem with this is that only eating junk food is just as risky as not eating at all.

Picky eaters can be a challenge at best; however, you may find that offering them raw juices and smoothies is something that they actually enjoy! Take a look at the following tips on juicing for picky eaters:

➢ There is probably at least one type of fruit your "picky eater" enjoys - introduce them to their juicing regimen by starting them out using juices made up of at least 80% of that favorite fruit. Once they become more willing to drink the juice, begin decreasing the percentage of their favorite fruit and begin increasing the percentage of other fruits, vegetables, and greens.

Another alternative is to start them off on one type of produce at a time – *only* one, not a mixture of multiple types of produce – and give them a small amount of juice at a time, such as one-half cup. Great types of produce that taste great solo include apples, oranges, and watermelon. Mix the fruit with one-part water. For sweeter fruits such as pears, grapes, and cherries, mix with two-parts water. Once your child gets used to these one-fruit raw juices, you can begin to mix in other types of fruits, then eventually vegetables and greens.

➢ Take your "picky eater" to the store and tell them to pick out a special cup that they can use *only* for juicing. Your child will feel like a part of the juicing process and will look at their chosen cup and juicing as a very special thing. This may not work as well for older kids, but it works wonders on children ages 8 and below!

➢ Let your "picky eater" taste test different fruits and vegetables and choose what type of produce they want their juice to made with. This will help to give them some control over what they are putting into their mouths.

➢ When you offer your "picky eater" his juice, say nothing. Do not make any comment. Don't tell him about how good the juice is for him, or that it's healthy, or anything. Hand him his juice in the same manner you would hand him a glass of water. Don't make a big deal out of it, and neither will your picky eater!

➢ If you offer your "picky eater" the juice and she refuses it, don't fuss or argue. Take it away and let the matter go – but don't let her think she has won! Try to give her the juice again in a day or two. If she refuses, then let it go again without comment. Keep trying to re-introduce the juice until that picky eater finally gives in. Once that happens, celebrate and shower her with tons of compliments and praise!

➢ Try to get your "picky eater's" siblings to drink their juices nearby and show how much they thoroughly enjoy them. You too, mom and dad! Your picky eater is constantly watching what you choose to eat and not eat! Set a good example by showing your picky eater how much you love juice as well!

➤ Popsicles! Juice your fruit, and even vegetables, and freeze them into ice cube trays with popsicle sticks or by using popsicle molds. This is an excellent way to get your picky eater to begin their juicing regimen. Kids love popsicles! Another option is to make your picky eater a smoothie instead of raw juice. The nutrients are the same, yet kids would choose icy smoothies over straight juice any day!

Daily Juicing Intake for Children

Let's take a look at the appropriate daily juicing intake according to the age of your child. **Note:** You know your child best, so use this only as a suggestion and follow your parental instinct. You may feel your child needs more or less juice than the amounts listed below:

Ages 0 to 2: Children under two years of age, particularly those who are breastfed, typically do not need to be on a juicing regimen. Most kids do not need to begin a juicing regimen until they begin to be introduced to processed foods and worldly toxins, such as when they begin eating solid foods, start school, begin playing outdoors, etc.

Ages 3 to 5: Begin their daily juicing regimen with ¼ cup, diluted with one-part water. When they can comfortably drink the juice on a steady basis, you can increase the amount to 1/3 cup - always remember to dilute the juice with water. This age range of children can safely be on a juicing regimen of ¼ to 1/3 cup (2- to 3-ounces) 1 to 3 times daily, depending on how well their bodies take the raw juices. For this age group, keep each juice to a maximum of 1/3 of a cup. That isn't that much juice – but the benefits that little amount holds are enormous! Most 3 year-olds do well at ¼ cup twice daily. 4 and 5 year-olds tend to do better at 1/3 cup 2 to 3 times daily.

Ages 6 to 8: If your child is starting a juicing regimen for the first time, begin by offering them

½ cup of juice, diluted with one-part water, 2 to 4 times daily. Continue diluting the juices with water for the first 2 to 3 weeks of the regimen. If your child has been on a juicing regimen for at least 6 months, begin with ½ cup of raw juice but DO NOT dilute with water. At this age, your child will do fine with straight juice. Once your child has been on a steady regimen for some time, you can increase the amount to ¾ cup juice 2 to 4 times daily.

Ages: 9 to 12: 9 to 12 year-olds can start out 1 cup (8-ounces) of raw juice (if your child is new to juicing, dilute with one-part water for the first 1 to 2 weeks) 2 to 5 times daily. When your child is on a steady regimen, you can increase the amount of juice to a maximum of 1¼ cups (10-ounces) 2 to 5 times daily.

Ages 13 and Up: At this age, water dilution is not necessary. This age group can safely drink 1 to 1½ cups (8- to 12-ounces) of raw juice 3 to 5 times daily.

Let's move on to chapter 5, where we can start looking at some of the best fruits and vegetables to offer your children as a part of their juicing regimen!

CHAPTER 5: JUICING FRUITS AND VEGETABLES

The Best Produce to Juice for Kids:

If your kids are new to juicing, start by juicing fruits and vegetables that you know they enjoy. Perhaps your daughter loves apples or your son loves watermelon. There are some beginner juicers who beg their parents for carrot juice mixed with a bit of a sweet fruit or tomato. Cucumber juice is another favorite among children who are new to juicing.

Beginner juicers tend to prefer cold and sweet juices. It is a good idea to pour their juice over ice. When they become more advanced in their juicing regimen, they will be able to better tolerate juice at room temperature or juice that has a slightly blander taste.

Remember, it is important to drink the juice immediately after juicing so that your child gains the maximum amount of nutrients. When you allow juices to sit, even for a couple of minutes, the juice will begin to quickly lose nutrients. Many people think that it's okay to make the juice and then place it in the freezer to chill. This will only leave you with trace amounts of nutrients. You should encourage you kids to drink their juice within 10 minutes of offering it to them.

Always start out with mild fruits and vegetables that are calm on the stomach such as carrots, apples, grapes, pears, watermelon, cucumber, and tomatoes. Try juicing one fruit or vegetable at a time. When your kids get used to solo fruit juices, you can begin to mix in other fruits and vegetables.

Once your child has been on a steady juicing regimen for about 3 to 4 weeks, you can begin adding in other items to boost up the nutrients such as edible weeds, flax seed, and ground nuts and seeds. There is really no limit to the things you can juice. Have fun with it!

"The Dirty Dozen" and "The Clean 15"

Each year, the Environmental Working Group, which consists of researchers, scientists, and policymakers, comes together to compile two lists. One list consists of produce that contain the highest amounts of pesticides, otherwise known as "The Dirty Dozen." The second list is of produce that has proven to hold the lowest amount of pesticides. This list is referred to as "The Clean 15."

The Dirty Dozen list refers to 12 different fruits and vegetables that you should always buy organic. It is said that buying organic produce can reduce the amount of toxins your body takes in by up to 80%. The fruits and vegetables on the 2012 Dirty Dozen list tested positive for between 40 to 70 different toxic chemicals – *yuck*!

There is also new list referred to as "The Dirty Dozen Plus" which now includes two types of produce that have been teetering on the verge of being a part of the Dirty Dozen list. Because they were always a few points behind the top twelve, they weren't added until recently. The Environmental Working Group now considers them to be a valid part of the Dirty Dozen and has thus adopted the new "Dirty Dozen Plus" list.

NOTE: It's always better to spend those extra pennies on organic produce, rather than knowing that toxic chemicals are being consumed by your children.

The Clean 15, on the other hand, refer to 15 different fruits and vegetables which you don't have to worry about buying organic. These fruits and vegetables showed little to no trace of pesticides and other chemicals. Save your money and pick up the regular versions with a clear conscience.

The Dirty Dozen Plus and Clean 15 Lists for 2012 are as follows:

"The Dirty Dozen Plus" 2012

1. Apples
2. Celery
3. Sweet Bell Peppers
4. Peaches
5. Strawberries
6. Imported Nectarines
7. Grapes
8. Spinach
9. Lettuce
10. Cucumbers
11. Domestic Blueberries
12. Potatoes
13. Green Beans
14. Kale, Collards, and Leafy Greens

"The Clean 15" 2012

1. Onions
2. Sweet Corn
3. Pineapple
4. Avocado
5. Cabbage
6. Sweet Peas
7. Asparagus
8. Mangoes
9. Eggplant

10. Kiwi
11. Domestic Cantaloupe
12. Sweet Potatoes
13. Grapefruit
14. Watermelon
15. Mushrooms

Selecting Fresh Produce

When shopping for fresh fruits and vegetables at your local farmer's market, grocery store, or picking them out of your garden, you always want to pick the cream of the crop.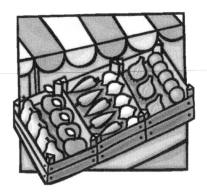

You want to be picky about picking out your produce! There are some general guidelines that should always be followed when it comes to selecting produce. They are as follows:

 If you are picking your own produce, be sure to bring along clean bags or containers.

 Handle the produce very gently to reduce the risk of any bruising or damage caused by handling. If you are at the supermarket, be sure to keep produce at the top of the shopping cart. Careful; don't allow other foods to lie on top of the produce. Also, be sure to keep your fruits and vegetables away from any fresh meats that are also in the cart. Don't be a drill sergeant, but make sure that the checkout clerk and employee bagging your groceries also handle the produce with care. You could choose to bag the produce yourself, to ensure safe packing.

 Look for fruits and vegetables that are free from signs of mold or other types of spoilage. Also refrain from selecting produce if it has foul or unusual odors or colors.

 Buying fruits and vegetables that are not yet ripe to take home and store until they ripen is not always a good idea. Some produce such as nectarines and peaches will often soften during storage, but they won't ripen.

 When buying produce that is pre-cut, always be sure that it has been, and is, properly refrigerated. Continue to keep it cold during transport, even if you need to bring a cooler along with you in the car. If you use a cooler, fill it with ice packs – like the frozen ice packs used in children's lunch boxes, these work wonders for keeping produce at the right temperature for the ride home. Regular ice cubes will melt which can result in the produce becoming soggy.

Selecting Fresh Vegetables	
VEGETABLE	**SELECTION PROCESS**
Artichoke	Hold the artichoke in your hand; it should have a thick and firm feel about it when you gently squeeze it. Try breaking off a leaf or two – the leaves should snap off into your hand cleanly and with little effort when pulled. Avoid artichokes that have brown and/or separated leaves.
Arugula, raw	Select fresh arugula that has long, firm, bright green leaves. Avoid any holes, wilting, or yellowing.
Asparagus	The stalks should be tender and firm. The tips of the asparagus should be close and packed in. Try to find asparagus with the least amount of white as possible. The less white the asparagus, the tenderer it is. Asparagus toughens quickly, so only buy or pick the amount you are planning on using that same day.
Bell Pepper	Choose bell peppers that have smooth skin with no bruises or marks on the surface.
Bok Choy	The best bok choy has flared, jungle-green leafy blades and the stalks should be thick, translucent, and white in color. The stalks should be firm.
Broccoli	The buds should be green and tightly closed, The stalks should not be taut and the florets should be a dark, deep green in color. Avoid buying/picking broccoli with yellowing leaves and a strong odor.
Brussels Sprouts	The flower clusters should be tight and close together. Avoid selecting those with smudges or dirty spots, which could indicate pest or disease presence.
Butternut Squash	The squash should feel firm and heavy for its size. Tap on the squash with your knuckles, it should sound hollow. The squash should have firm and smooth skin, not flaky, peeling or dented skin.
Cabbage	Select cabbage heads that are compact and firm. The leaves should be fresh and crispy. The leaves should not have any markings or brown spots. The head of cabbage should only have a few loose outer leaves, the darker green the leaves, the more flavor the cabbage has.
Carrots	Select firm, plump carrots with roots and leaves that are healthy-looking and brightly colored. Avoid selecting carrots with cracks in the skin. Carrots containing smaller cores are typically sweeter and better tasting. Since you are not able to actually see the core until you cut into the carrot, select carrots that are thinner and smaller at the top – these are common indicators of small cores.
Cauliflower	You want a clean, creamy-white, tight curd. The bud clusters should be tight with no separation. The clusters should not be dull in color or spotted. Look for heads of cauliflower that are surrounded by green leaves, as the cauliflower will be fresher and will have been better protected.
Cucumber	Select cucumbers that are medium to dark green in color. They should feel firm when squeezed. Their skin should be firm and tough, not soft, wrinkled/wilted.

Eggplant	Select an eggplant that has glossy skin. Press the eggplant with your finger and let go, there should be a little indentation mark left behind from your finger, but it should immediately bounce back to form.
Green Beans	Choose green beans that are slender and crisp - making a "snap" sound when broken in half. The beans should be brightly colored and have no blemishes.
Jicama	Select tubers that are plump and heavy for their size, the skin should be either smooth or rough to the touch. The skin color should be uniform; it is okay if there is minimal blotchiness, as it won't affect the flesh underneath, Avoid selecting jicama with bruising or any signs of mold. Avoid any damage, cuts, and soft spots in the skin as well.
Kale	Select kale which has hardy stems that are moist and firm with deeply-colored leaves.
Spaghetti Squash	The rind should be even yellow to orange in color. The squash should be firm and heavy. It should not puncture when poked.
Spinach, raw	Select spinach with dark green, crispy leaves. The spinach should have a nice, fresh fragrance. Avoid spinach that has leaves which are limp, damaged, or spotted.
Tomatillo	Select tomatillos that are smooth and sticky to the touch and yellowish-green in color. They should feel firmer than a ripe tomato, but still slightly soft to the touch.
Tomato	Tomatoes should be soft with firm skin when pressed, but not mushy. They should have a distinct fresh aroma. Avoid selecting tomatoes that have bruises, blemishes, or discolorations.
Winter Squash	Look for a tough, hard rind. The squash should be heavy for its size.
Yams	Select yams which do not have any cracks or soft spots. Yams should feel firm and offer a little give when squeezed.
Zucchini	A ripe zucchini should have a firm, but not soft, texture. They should be the same shade of green all over, and feel slightly flexible when handled. Avoid signs of decay, such as cuts, sunken spots, punctures, and/or moldy spots

Selecting Fresh Fruits	
FRUIT	**SELECTION PROCESS**
Apple	The apple should be firm to the touch. There should not be any mushy or soft areas. Avoid selecting apples that have discolorations and brown spots.
Apricots	The deeper orange colored the apricots are, the more nutrient rich they are. Choose apricots that are slightly soft, yet firm.
Avocado	The avocado should be soft when gently squeezed, but not so much that it feels loose under the skin.
Banana	Choose bananas that are solid yellow in color, avoid bananas that have bruising or soft spots. A banana should be firm with a little give, but not soft. This is one fruit where it is okay to buy pre-ripened when they are green and ripen at home. The best way to ripen bananas at home is to place them in a brown paper bag. Remember: Green = Under-ripe; Yellow = Ripe; Brown = Over-ripe.
Berries	No matter whether you are selecting blueberries, blackberries, raspberries, strawberries or any other type of berries – you want to select berries that are plump and solid with vibrant colors. Don't buy berries if their container is stained as it means the berries are leaky and weak. You want berries that hold their juices inside of them. If berries have clinging caps, it probably means that they are not yet completely ripe.
Cantaloupe	The stem "eye" should smell sweet. Push the stem "eye" with your finger, it should give a little when pushed, but it should not be mushy. A perfect cantaloupe has a golden-yellow outer skin. Avoid selecting cantaloupe which is too green.
Cherimoya	To select a ripe cherimoya, take it in your hands and gently squeeze it. There should be a little give when squeezed. When squeezing it, you may feel like it will burst or puncture when pressed.
Cherries	Select firm red cherries with the stems attached. Avoid cherries which are too soft, too shriveled, or those that are blemished.
Coconut	Select a coconut that feels heavy for its size. Shake the coconut; it should sound as if it is full of liquid; the more liquid, the better the coconut.
Dragon Fruit	The skin should be bright and evenly colored all over. Avoid dragon fruit that is covered in brown spots. The leaves should look healthy and be in good condition. When you squeeze this fruit, it should be firm and not soft or mushy.
Fig	Select figs that are very mushy and soft, so much so that if you squeezed them too hard, the insides should fall out.
Grapefruit	Select grapefruit that are a deep yellow-orange in color. The fruit should be firm to the touch and have thick and springy skin.
Grapes	Select grapes which are firm and vibrant in color. Grapes which are soft or feel like tiny water balloons are usually too ripe.
Guava	Select guava that is yellow, white, or reddish in color. Avoid selecting a guava that has too much green coloring. A ripe guava is mushy and easily dented by your finger when pushing the skin.

Honeydew Melon	Perfect honeydew should feel heavy for its size. It should not be at all mushy or soft, nor should it be too hard or firm. The stem "eye" should be sweet smelling and offer a slight give when pushed in with thumb.
Kiwi	Select kiwi that is not too mushy or soft when pushed with your finger. The skin should be taut, smooth, and have no wrinkles.
Kumquat	Select kumquats that are bright-orange in color, well-shaped, and firm to the touch. Avoid any soft spots.
Lemon	A ripe lemon is completely yellow with no green tint. Over-ripe lemons begin to brown in color.
Lime	Choose limes which are a nicely colored green. Choose limes which are firm, but offer a little give when squeezed. Avoid markings, bruising, etc.
Mango	Select mangoes that are squishy to the touch, but not overly soft. Select a mango that smells citrusy and fruity.
Nectarine	Select nectarines that are soft when you squeeze them, but not mushy – they should be a deep red - its okay if there is yellow, as well.
Orange	Select oranges that are firm and heavy for their size. Their skin should be smooth and free of any brown spots. Pick oranges which are deep orange in color for juicier fruit.
Papaya	A ripe papaya will have skin that is shaded as if it is turning green to yellow in color. A little bruising is okay, but a lot is not. The papaya should not be either mushy or sweet smelling; this indicates that it may be over-ripe.
Passion Fruit	Pick passion fruit that are dimpled and dark purple in appearance. When you pick them up, they should feel heavy.
Peach	Peaches should be yellowish-red with firm, smooth, and velvety thin skin. They should be bruise and blemish-free and not have any soft or mushy spots. They should not be hard – there should be some give when squeezed.
Pear	Select pears that are firm but not hard. Press your finger near the stem, there should be a little give. Pick pears that do not have dark splotches or very soft spots.
Persimmon	Select this fruit if the skin is deeply-red in color, free from any blemishes, with glossy skin.
Pineapple	Look at the "eyes" located at the base of the pineapple; they should have a golden yellow color (the higher the golden yellow rises up the base of the fruit, the more ripe the pineapple). The pineapple should smell sweet and feel firm, not overly soft.
Plantain	Select plantains that are dark brown to black in color – they should yield to pressure and feel very mushy – that's good!
Plum	A ripe plum will yield to a gentle amount of pressure. A plum that is too hard may not be able to ripen fully on its own. They should be deep purple to black in color depending on the variety of plum.
Star Fruits	These fruits should be bright yellow with as few green spots as possible. There may be a few brown spots, but not excessive. They should be firm to the touch and not at all mushy.
Watermelon	Ripe watermelons are dull in color but their outer skin is shiny. Squeeze the watermelon and listen for movement and/or cracking inside – this is good and signifies that the

	watermelon is ripe and ready, There should also be some external yellow color to one side – this also indicates ripeness.

Storing Fresh Fruits and Vegetables

Knowing how to properly store fresh fruits and vegetables if they are not to be used right away is just as important in knowing how to select quality produce. Storing produce the correct way is not as simple as you may think. Certain conditions can affect the way fresh fruits and vegetables are preserved in storage. There are a number of factors that can influence whether or not fresh produce is stored properly. Some of these factors include temperature, humidity, and atmospheric ethylene, among others.

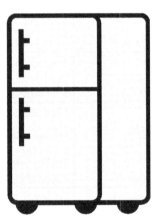

Each variety of fruit and vegetables have their own requirements for being stored. Since the proper storage of food varies greatly per type of produce, there are really no general guidelines. There are a few golden "rules" however that should be followed when preparing to store fresh produce, they are as follows:

Quick Tips and Suggestions for Storing Fresh Produce

 Fresh fruits and vegetables should be eaten as soon as possible, so that you get the most nutrition and flavor.

 Seasonal conditions can influence or dictate different storage methods for fresh produce. Pay attention to storing guidelines in your area.

 You can store most perishable fruits and vegetables in the refrigerator at a temperature of 40° F or below. All produce that is purchased as pre-cut or peeled MUST be stored in the refrigerator.

 Don't wash vegetables before refrigerating, but rather wash before eating. Too much moisture is detrimental.

 For produce items that must be stored at room temperature, make sure that they are not stored in direct sunlight. A great option is to use a perforated plastic bag.

 All fruit that is ripe must be stored in the refrigerator.

 The average longevity of stored produce is 1 to 2 weeks. Make sure the produce is consumed before then, so you don't end up throwing anything away.

 When storing produce in drawers in the refrigerator, keep fruits and veggies separate as ethylene can easily build up in the fridge and cause spoilage.

 When storing herbs, snip off the ends and place them to store upright in a glass of water. Cover the glass with a plastic bag.

Take a look at the following tables to get information of proper storage guidelines for individual types of fruits and vegetables.

Storing Fresh Vegetables

VEGETABLE	STORAGE GUIDELINES
Artichoke	Store in the refrigerator, wrapped in plastic, for no more than 1 to 2 weeks.
Asparagus	Store in the refrigerator, wrapped in plastic, for no more than 4 days.
Beets	Store in the refrigerator, greens removed, wrapped in plastic, for up to 2 weeks.
Bell Pepper	Store in the refrigerator (no colder than 40° F) in plastic, for no more than 1 week.
Bok Choy	Store in the refrigerator, wrapped in plastic, for no more than 4 days.
Broccoli	Store in the refrigerator, wrapped in plastic, for no more than 5 days.
Brussels Sprouts	Store in the refrigerator, wrapped in plastic, for no more than 5 days - flavor gets stronger over time.
Butternut Squash	Store in a cool, dry, well-ventilated place, unwrapped, for up to 1 month.
Cabbage	Store in the refrigerator, tightly wrapped in plastic, for up to 2 weeks.
Carrots	Store in the refrigerator, greens removed, wrapped in plastic for up to 3 weeks.
Cauliflower	Store in the refrigerator, wrapped in plastic, for no more than 1 week.
Celery	Store in the refrigerator (no colder than 40° F) in a vented plastic bag, for up to 2 weeks.
Collard Greens	Store in the refrigerator, wrapped in plastic, for no more than 5 days.
Cucumber	Store in the refrigerator, wrapped in plastic, for no more than 1 week.
Dandelion Greens	Store in the refrigerator, in a plastic bag, for 1 to 2 days.
Eggplant	Store in the refrigerator (no colder than 40° F) in a vented plastic or paper bag, for up to 5 days.
Fennel	Store in the refrigerator, in plastic, for up to 5 days.
Garlic	Store in a cool, dry, well-ventilated place, unwrapped, for up to 2 months for whole bulbs and 10 days for cloves.
Ginger Root	Store in the refrigerator, wrapped in dry paper towel and placed in plastic, for 2 to 3 weeks.
Green Beans	Store in the refrigerator, in plastic bag with dry paper towel, for up to 7 days.

Green Onions	Store in the refrigerator's vegetable crisper, in plastic, for 7 to 10 days.
Herbs, fresh	Store in the refrigerator, wrapped in slightly damp paper towel and placed in plastic, for 3 to 7 days - depending on the type of herb.
Jicama	Store in the refrigerator, wrapped in plastic, for up to 3 weeks. For cut jicama: store in the refrigerator, wrapped tightly in plastic, for up to 1 week.
Kale	Store in the refrigerator, wrapped in plastic, for no more than 5 days.
Kohlrabi	Store in the refrigerator, in a plastic bag, for 4 to 5 days.
Lettuce, Bibb	Store in the refrigerator, in a loosely closed plastic bag, for up to 1 week.
Lettuce, Boston	Store in the refrigerator, in a loosely closed plastic bag, for up to 1 week.
Lettuce, Butterhead	Store in the refrigerator, in a loosely closed plastic bag, for up to 1 week.
Lettuce, Bagged/Prewashed	Store in the refrigerator, in the closed bag or tied bag, for 7 to 10 days or by date on bag.
Lettuce, Iceberg	Store in the refrigerator, in a loosely closed plastic bag, for up to 1 week.
Lettuce, Leaf	Store in the refrigerator, in a loosely closed plastic bag, for up to 1 week.
Lettuce, Romaine	Store in the refrigerator, in a loosely closed plastic bag, for up to 1 week.
Onion (white, yellow)	Store in a cool, dry, well-ventilated place, unwrapped, for 2 weeks to 2 months - depending on the variety.
Rhubarb	Store in the refrigerator, in plastic, for up to 7 days.
Snap Peas (sugar, snap, or snow)	Store in the refrigerator, wrapped in plastic, for 5 to 7 days.
Spaghetti Squash	Store in a cool, dry, well-ventilated place, unwrapped, for up to 1 month.
Spinach, raw	Store in the refrigerator, in plastic wrapped in dry paper towel, for no more than 7 days.
Summer Squash	Store in a cool, dry, well-ventilated place, wrapped in plastic, for up to 5 days.
Swiss Chard	Store in the refrigerator, wrapped in plastic, for no more than 5 days.
Tomatillo	Store at room temperature, unwrapped, for up to 5 days.
Tomato	Store at room temperature, unwrapped, for up to 5 days.

Watercress	Store in the refrigerator, with stems wrapped in damp paper towel and placed in plastic bag, for 2 to 3 days.
Winter Squash	Store in a cool, dry, well-ventilated place, unwrapped, for up to 1 month.
Yams	Store in a cool, dry, well-ventilated place, unwrapped, for 1 to 4 weeks.
Zucchini	Store in a cool, dry, well-ventilated place, wrapped in plastic, for up to 5 days.

FRUITS	STORAGE GUIDELINES
Apple	Store in the refrigerator, unwrapped, for up to 3 weeks.
Apricots	Ripen at room temperature. Once ripe, store in the refrigerator, unwrapped, for 4 to 5 days.
Avocado	Ripen at room temperature, unwrapped, then refrigerate, wrapped, for up to 4 days.
Bananas	Ripen at room temperature, unwrapped; if overripe, refrigerate for 2 days (skin will blacken).
Berries (Raspberries, Blackberries, Boysenberries)	Refrigerate in vented container for up to 3 days.
Blueberries	Refrigerate in vented container for up to 4 days.
Cantaloupe	Ripen at room temperature, unwrapped, then refrigerate for up to 5 days. If cut, store in the refrigerator, wrapped in plastic, for up to 3 days.
Casaba Melon	Ripen at room temperature, unwrapped, then refrigerate for up to 5 days. If cut, store in refrigerator, wrapped in plastic, for up to 3 days.
Cherimoya	Ripen at room temperature. Once ripe, store in refrigerator, unwrapped, for up to 2 days.
Cherries	Store in refrigerator, wrapped in plastic, for up to 5 days.
Coconut	Store at room temperature or in the refrigerator, unwrapped, for up to 1 month; If cut, store in the refrigerator, in coconut juice or water, for up to 1 week.
Cranberries	Store in the refrigerator, in a plastic bag or covered container, for up to 1 month.
Dragon Fruit	Store in the refrigerator, unwrapped, for 2 to 3 days.
Fig	Store in the refrigerator, in a plastic bag, for up to 2 days. May be frozen for up to 2 months.
Grapefruit	Store at room temperature, unwrapped, for 1 week, or store in the refrigerator for 2 weeks.
Grapes	Store in the refrigerator, in a vented plastic bag, for up to 1 week.
Guava	Ripen at room temperature, unwrapped, then refrigerate, in a plastic bag, for up to 4 days.
Honeydew Melon	Ripen at room temperature, unwrapped, then refrigerate for up to 5 days. If cut, store in the refrigerator, wrapped in plastic, for up to 3 days.
Kiwi	Ripen at room temperature, unwrapped, then refrigerate for up to 4 days.
Lemon	Store at room temperature, unwrapped, for 1 week OR store in the refrigerator for 2 weeks.
Lime	Store at room temperature, unwrapped, for 1 week OR store in the refrigerator for 2 weeks.
Mango	Ripen at room temperature, unwrapped, then refrigerate for up to 1 week.
Nectarine	Ripen at room temperature, unwrapped, then refrigerate, in vented plastic bag, for 4

	days.
Orange	Store at room temperature, unwrapped, for 1 week OR store in the refrigerator for 2 weeks.
Papaya	Ripen at room temperature, unwrapped, then refrigerate for up to 1 week.
Passion Fruit	Ripen at room temperature, unwrapped, then refrigerate for 5 to 7 days.
Peaches	Ripen at room temperature, unwrapped, then refrigerate, in a vented plastic bag, for 4 days.
Pear	Ripen at room temperature, unwrapped, then refrigerate for up to 4 days.
Persimmon	Ripen at room temperature, unwrapped, then refrigerate in a plastic bag, for 2 to 3 days. If cut up, wrap tightly in aluminum foil or plastic wrap, place in an air-tight container, and refrigerate for up to 4 days.
Pineapple	Store in the refrigerator, unwrapped, for up to 5 days. If cut, store in the refrigerator, tightly wrapped in plastic, for up to 3 days.
Plantain	If whole, ripen at room temperature, unwrapped, then refrigerate for 3 to 5 days. If cut up, wrap tightly in aluminum foil or plastic wrap, place in an air-tight container and refrigerate for up to 4 days.
Plum	Ripen at room temperature, unwrapped, then refrigerate for up to 4 days.
Pomegranates	Store at room temperature, unwrapped, for 1 to 2 weeks OR store in the refrigerator, unwrapped, for up to 2 months.
Star Fruits	Ripen at room temperature, unwrapped, then refrigerate for 5 to 7 days.
Strawberries	Store in refrigerator, in vented container, for up to 3 days.
Tangerines	Store at room temperature, unwrapped, for 1 week OR store in the refrigerator for 2 weeks.
Tomatillo	Store at room temperature, unwrapped, for up to 5 days.
Tomato	Store at room temperature, unwrapped, for up to 5 days.
Ugli Fruit	Store at room temperature for up to 1 week OR store in the refrigerator, in a plastic bag, for up to 2 weeks.
Watermelon	Store at room temperature, unwrapped, for 4 days OR store in the refrigerator for 2 weeks. If cut up, store in the refrigerator, wrapped in plastic, for up to 3 days.

Learning how to properly store fruits and veggies will save you quite a bit of money if you do it the right way, and you do it consistently. Store your produce well to extend its shelf life, so you can get the absolute most out of it!

• • •

How to Juice: From Prep to Juicer

Now you know which types of produce to select for your child's juicing regimen. You're practically an expert on how to select and store fresh produce to get the most out of it. Let's now discuss the steps you should take in moving the selected fruits and vegetables from the grocery bag to the juicer. The process is simple, and once you have it down, you will be amazed by how convenient and easy it is to offer your kids something that is so powerfully nutritious! Let's get started...

Now that you have picked out some delicious fruits and vegetables, it's time to prepare them for juicing. Basic guidelines you should always follow in preparing your produce and juicing machine for juicing include:

- Thoroughly wash ALL produce before juicing to remove any pesticide build-up! There are produce washing fluids available at most grocery and health food stores, but rinsing vigorously with cool water is just as useful.

- Be sure to cut away and discard any bruised or damages areas on produce.

- Always remove the peels of grapefruits, oranges, and tangerines before juicing. The skins of these fruits are very bitter and can wreak havoc on one's digestive system. Lemon and lime peels can be juiced ONLY if they are organic, but they can add an unappealing flavor to your juice. It is important to leave as much of the white, stringy-filmy part of these citrus fruits as possible as it is loaded with bioflavonoids and vitamin C. The peels of papayas and mangoes MUST be peeled away and discarded as they contain an irritant with can be harmful in frequent consumption. A good rule-of-thumb to follow is to remove the peels and skins of all produce unless it is organic.

- Remove any hard seeds, pits, and stones from produce such as peaches, plums, and cherries. Softer seeds such as those from watermelon, cucumbers, grapes, and oranges can be juiced without concern. Apple seeds are best avoided, as they contain cyanides and arsenic that can be toxic when too much is consumed.

- The stems and leaves of most produce CAN and SHOULD be juiced. There are many nutrients available in the leaves and stems of many different types of produce. However, thicker grape stems can dull juicer blades, and the greens from rhubarb and carrots should *always* be removed and discarded as they contain toxic substances.

- Cut produce in chunks that will easily fit through your juicer's feeding tube. Trying to cram too large of produce down the feeding tube will eventually destroy your juicer. Remember, the larger the feed tube, the bigger the sections of produce that can be fed into the juicer.

- Remember that some types of produce do not juice as well as others. A good guideline to follow is the more water a fruit or veggie contains the easier it is to juice. The less water produce contains, the harder it is to juice. Some examples of produce that do not juice as well include avocados, bananas, and coconut. It is important when processing these types of produce to first juice the watery produce. Then transfer the extracted juice into a blender and blend the hard-to-juice produce with the extracted juices.

- The MOST important guideline to follow is to encourage your children to drink their juices as soon as possible in order for them to benefit the most from the vitamins and minerals. Light, heat, and air can very quickly kill nutrients! It is crucial that if you are unable to consume juices immediately, you should store them in the fridge for no longer than 24 hours in airtight and opaque containers. Remember: the longer a juice sits → the more oxidized it becomes → the more nutrients are lost. So get those kiddos to DRINK UP!!!

Now it's time to experiment with some kid-friendly juicing recipes! Part 2 is compiled of a handful of recipes that kids are sure to love!

Kid-Friendly

Juicing Recipes

CHAPTER 6: KID-FRIENDLY JUICING RECIPES

In this section, we will take a look at some recipes that your kids will not only love, but that will also help in getting your children on a steady juicing regimen. All of these juices are made up of fruit and vegetable combinations that will help your child's body adjust to fresh fruits and vegetables in a safe way.

Remember, when starting your children on a juicing regimen, it is important to start them on fresh fruit and vegetable juices made up of one type of fruit or vegetable. After one week of a steady regimen, you can begin to combine two different types of fruits and vegetables. After week 3, begin combining three or more fruits and vegetables. This will give your child's body the time it needs to adjust.

The recipes in this section will first take you through the first four weeks of your child's introductory juicing regimen. Keep in mind that the first four weeks of recipes are meant for those kids who are brand new to juicing. If your child has been juicing for some time, then you can either skip ahead or feel free to use these beginner recipes anyway! After the first four weeks of recipes, we will begin to look at different recipes that are designed to meet specific needs of your child, such as recipes that will help your child recover quickly from the common cold.

Again, you know your child better than anyone, so while these recipes are here as a guide, use your best judgment in the appropriate combinations of produce for your child.

NOTE: *The nutrition info listed is only an estimate. The actual data will vary depending on exact amount given to child, the different types of produce used, and so on.*

Juicing Regimen for Kids – Week One

Week one's recipes consist of single fruits or vegetables. The recipes are simple; your child should accept these juices fairly willingly.

Juicing Regimen for Kids: Week One - Day One

Apple Juice

Juice prep to finish: 4 minutes

Difficulty: Easy

Yield: (2) 4 oz. (125ml) cup

Ingredients:

- ⍦ 2 to 3 medium apples of choice, skinned and sliced (make sure all seeds are removed)
- ⍦ ¼ cup filtered water, to dilute (for kids under the age of 6)
- ⍦ Ice, optional

Instructions:

1. Wash and skin the apple. Cut into slices and make sure all seeds are removed.
2. Process the apple slices through juicer.
3. For kids under 6 years of age: Dilute with 1/4 cup water.
4. Pour juice into cup, over ice if desired.
5. Encourage your child to drink the juice immediately in order to benefit from all the nutrients. Any remaining juice can be refrigerated for up 48 hours, in an airtight, opaque container in order to reduce exposure to light, heat, or air due to risk of oxidation and loss of nutrients.

Nutritional info: ⍦ Calories: 97 ⍦ Total Fat: 0g ⍦ Total Carbohydrates: 22g ⍦ Dietary Fiber: 4g ⍦ Sugars: 32g ⍦ Protein: 0g ⍦ Sodium: 0mg

Juicing Regimen for Kids: Week One - Day Two

Orange Juice

Juice prep to finish: 4 minutes

Difficulty: Easy

Yield: (2) 4 oz. (125ml) cup

Ingredients:

- 1 to 1½ medium oranges of choice peeled and sectioned.
- ¼ cup filtered water, to dilute (for kids under the age of 6)
- Ice, optional

Instructions:

1. Wash and peel the oranges. Cut into slices and section.
2. Process the orange sections through juicer.
3. For kids under 6 years of age: Dilute with 1/4 cup water.
4. Pour juice into cup, over ice if desired.
5. Encourage your child to drink the juice immediately in order to benefit from all the nutrients. Any remaining juice can be refrigerated for up 48 hours, in an airtight, opaque container, so as to not be exposed to light, heat, or air due to risk of oxidation and loss of nutrients.

Nutritional info: Calories: 84 Total Fat: 0g Total Carbohydrates: 30g Dietary Fiber: 6g Sugars: 24g Protein: 2g Sodium: 0mg

Juicing Regimen for Kids: Week One - Day Three

Pear Juice

Juice prep to finish: 5 minutes

Difficulty: Easy

Yield: (2) 4 oz. (125ml) cup

Ingredients:

- 1 to 2 small pears, stems removed, washed and cut into chunks.
- ¾ cup filtered water, to dilute (for kids under the age of 6)
- Ice, optional

Instructions:

1. Remove any stems and wash well. Skin stays intact. Cut into chunks. Remove seeds.
2. Process the pear chunks through juicer.
3. For kids under 6 years of age: Dilute with 3/4 cup water.
4. Pour juice into cup, over ice if desired.
5. Encourage your child to drink the juice immediately in order to benefit from all the nutrients. Any remaining juice can be refrigerated for up 48 hours, in an airtight, opaque container as to not be exposed to light, heat, or air due to risk of oxidation and loss of nutrients.

Nutritional info: Calories: 72 Total Fat: 0g Total Carbohydrates: 23g Dietary Fiber: 2g Sugars: 21g Protein: 2g Sodium: 2mg

Watermelon Juice (Watermelon Water)

Juice prep to finish: 5 minutes

Difficulty: Easy

Yield: (2) 4 oz. (125ml) cups

Ingredients:

- Y 2 to 4 cups seedless watermelon, cut into chunks and rind discarded
- Y ¼ cup filtered water, to dilute (for kids under the age of 6)
- Y Ice, optional

Instructions:

1. Cut Watermelon from rind then cut into chunks to make 2 to 4 cups watermelon pieces.
2. Process the watermelon chunks through juicer.
3. For kids under 6 years of age: Dilute with 1/4 cup water.
4. Pour juice into cup, over ice if desired.
5. Encourage your child to drink the juice immediately in order to benefit from all the nutrients. Any remaining juice can be refrigerated for up 48 hours, in an airtight, opaque container as to not be exposed to light, heat, or air due to risk of oxidation and loss of nutrients.

Nutritional info: Y Calories: 92 Y Total Fat: 0g Y Total Carbohydrates: 24g Y Dietary Fiber: 2g Y Sugars: 20g Y Protein: 2g Y Sodium: 4mg

Juicing Regimen for Kids: Week One - Day Five

Cucumber Juice

Juice prep to finish: 4 minutes

Difficulty: Easy

Yield: (2) 4 oz. (125ml) cups

Ingredients:

- Ƴ 1 to 2 medium cucumbers, peeled only if desired, and cut into sections.
- Ƴ ¼ cup filtered water, to dilute (for kids under the age of 6)
- Ƴ Ice, optional

Instructions:

1. Wash cucumbers and peel if desired. It is safe to juice the skin, if you choose to do so. Cut into sections.
2. Process the cucumber sections through juicer.
3. For kids under 6 years of age: Dilute with 1/4 cup water.
4. Pour juice into cup, over ice if desired.
5. Encourage your child to drink the juice immediately in order to benefit from all the nutrients. Any remaining juice can be refrigerated for up 48 hours, in an airtight, opaque container as to not be exposed to light, heat, or air due to risk of oxidation and loss of nutrients.

Nutritional info: Ƴ Calories: 45 Ƴ Total Fat: 0g Ƴ Total Carbohydrates: 11g Ƴ Dietary Fiber: 2g Ƴ Sugars: 5g Ƴ Protein: 2g Ƴ Sodium: 6mg

Juicing Regimen for Kids: Week One - Day Six

Grape Juice

Juice prep to finish: 4 minutes

Difficulty: Easy

Yield: (2) 4 oz. (125ml) cups

Ingredients:

- 2 to 4 cups of Concord grapes, stems removed
- 3/4 cup filtered water, to dilute (for kids under the age of 6)
- Ice, optional

Instructions:

1. Wash grapes and make sure all stems are removed.
2. Process the grapes through juicer.
3. For kids under 6 years of age: dilute with 1/4 cup water.
4. Pour juice into ¾ cup, over ice if desired.
5. Encourage your child to drink the juice immediately in order to benefit from all the nutrients. Any remaining juice can be refrigerated for up 48 hours, in an airtight, opaque container as to not be exposed to light, heat, or air due to risk of oxidation and loss of nutrients.

Nutritional info: Calories: 74 Total Fat: 0g Total Carbohydrates: 22g Dietary Fiber: 2g Sugars: 20g Protein: 2g Sodium: 4mg

Juicing Regimen for Kids: Week One - Day Seven

Pineapple Juice

Juice prep to finish: 4 minutes

Difficulty: Easy

Yield: (2) 4 oz. (125ml) cups

Ingredients:

- 2 to 4 cups of pineapple, cut into chunks
- ¼ cup filtered water, to dilute (for kids under the age of 6)
- Ice, optional

Instructions:

1. Remove the rind and cut the pineapple into sections and then chunks until you have 2 to 4 cups of pineapple pieces.
2. Process the pineapple through juicer.
3. For kids under 6 years of age: dilute with 1/4 cup water.
4. Pour juice into cup, over ice if desired.
5. Encourage your child to drink the juice immediately in order to benefit from all the nutrients. Any remaining juice can be refrigerated for up 48 hours, in an airtight, opaque container as to not be exposed to light, heat, or air due to risk of oxidation and loss of nutrients.

Nutritional info: Calories: 64 Total Fat: 0g Total Carbohydrates: 19g Dietary Fiber: 2g Sugars: 32g Protein: 2g Sodium: 4mg

Juicing Regimen for Kids – Week Two

Week two's recipes combine two different types of fruits or vegetables. The recipes are still very simple and your child should, again, accept these juices fairly willingly.

Juicing Regimen for Kids: Week Two - Day One

Pineapple - Apple Juice

Juice prep to finish: 6 minutes

Difficulty: Easy

Yield: (2) 4 oz. (125ml) cups

Ingredients:

- ϒ 2 to 4 cups of pineapple, cut into chunks
- ϒ 2 to 3 medium apples of choice, skinned and sliced (make sure all seeds are removed
- ϒ ¼ cup filtered water, to dilute (for kids under the age of 6)
- ϒ Ice, optional

Instructions:
1. Remove the rind and cut the pineapple into sections and then chunks until you have 2 to 4 cups of pineapple pieces.
2. Wash and skin the apple. Cut into slices and make sure all seeds are removed.
3. Process the pineapple and apple through juicer.
4. For kids under 6 years of age: dilute with 1/4 cup water.
5. Pour juice into cup, over ice if desired.
6. Encourage your child to drink the juice immediately in order to benefit from all the nutrients. Any remaining juice can be refrigerated for up 48 hours, in an airtight, opaque container as to not be exposed to light, heat, or air due to risk of oxidation and loss of nutrients.

Nutritional info: ϒ Calories: 58 ϒ Total Fat: 0g ϒ Total Carbohydrates: 23g ϒ Dietary Fiber: 2g ϒ Sugars: 32g ϒ Protein: 2g ϒ Sodium: 4mg

Juicing Regimen for Kids: Week Two - Day Two

Cucumber - Watermelon Juice

Juice prep to finish: 6 minutes

Difficulty: Easy

Yield: (2) 4 oz. (125ml) cups

Ingredients:

- ⍦ 2 to 4 cups seedless watermelon, cut into chunks and rind discarded
- ⍦ 1 large cucumber, with skin intact
- ⍦ ¼ cup filtered water, to dilute (for kids under the age of 6)
- ⍦ Ice, optional

Instructions:

1. Cut watermelon from rind then cut into chunks to make 2 to 4 cups watermelon pieces.
2. Wash cucumber thoroughly. Cut into sections, keeping skin intact.
3. Process the watermelon and cucumber through juicer.
4. For kids under 6 years of age: dilute with 1/4 cup water.
5. Pour juice into cup, over ice if desired.
6. Encourage your child to drink the juice immediately in order to benefit from all the nutrients. Any remaining juice can be refrigerated for up 48 hours, in an airtight, opaque container as to not be exposed to light, heat, or air due to risk of oxidation and loss of nutrients.

Nutritional info: ⍦ Calories: 52 ⍦ Total Fat: 0g ⍦ Total Carbohydrates: 27g ⍦ Dietary Fiber: 3g ⍦ Sugars: 18g ⍦ Protein: 2g ⍦ Sodium: 3mg

Juicing Regimen for Kids: Week Two - Day Three

Orange - Carrot Juice

Juice prep to finish: 6 minutes

Difficulty: Easy

Yield: (2) 4 oz. (125ml) cups

Ingredients:

- 1 to 1½ medium oranges of choice peeled and sectioned
- 1 to 2 carrots, greens removed, ends chopped off and discarded
- ¼ cup filtered water, to dilute (for kids under the age of 6)
- Ice, optional

Instructions:

1. Peel oranges and cut into sections.
2. Scrub carrots thoroughly. Remove any greens and discard. Cut off each end and discard. Cut each carrot in half.
3. Process the orange sections and carrots through juicer.
4. For kids under 6 years of age: Dilute with 1/4 cup water.
5. Pour juice into cup, over ice if desired.
6. Encourage your child to drink the juice immediately in order to benefit from all the nutrients. Any remaining juice can be refrigerated for up 48 hours, in an airtight, opaque container as to not be exposed to light, heat, or air due to risk of oxidation and loss of nutrients.

Nutritional info: Calories: 76 Total Fat: 0g Total Carbohydrates: 24g Dietary Fiber: 4g Sugars: 19g Protein: 3g Sodium: 25mg

Juicing Regimen for Kids: Week Two - Day Four

Cucumber - Apple Juice

Juice prep to finish: 6 minutes

Difficulty: Easy

Yield: (2) 4 oz. (125ml) cups

Ingredients:

- Υ 1 to 2 medium cucumbers, peeled only if desired, and cut into sections.
- Υ 2 to 3 medium apples of choice, skinned and sliced - make sure all seeds are removed.
- Υ ¼ cup filtered water, to dilute (for kids under the age of 6).
- Υ Ice, optional

Instructions:

1. Wash cucumbers and peel if desired. It is safe to juice the skin, if you choose to do so. Cut into sections.
2. Wash and skin the apple. Cut into slices and make sure all seeds are removed.
3. Process the cucumber and apple through juicer.
4. For kids under 6 years of age: Dilute with 1/4 cup water.
5. Pour juice into cup, over ice if desired.
6. Encourage your child to drink the juice immediately in order to benefit from all the nutrients. Any remaining juice can be refrigerated for up 48 hours, in an airtight, opaque container as to not be exposed to light, heat, or air due to risk of oxidation and loss of nutrients.

Nutritional info: Υ Calories: 52 Υ Total Fat: 0g Υ Total Carbohydrates: 12g Υ Dietary Fiber: 2g Υ Sugars: 29g Υ Protein: 2g Υ Sodium: 0mg

Juicing Regimen for Kids: Week Two - Day Five

Pineapple - Carrot Juice

Juice prep to finish: 6 minutes

Difficulty: Easy

Yield: (2) 4 oz. (125ml) cups

Ingredients:

- 2 to 4 cups of pineapple, cut into chunks
- 1 to 2 carrots, greens removed, ends chopped off and discarded
- ¼ cup filtered water, to dilute (for kids under the age of 6)
- Ice, optional

Instructions:

1. Remove the rind and cut the pineapple into sections and then chunks until you have 2 to 4 cups of pineapple pieces.
2. Scrub carrots thoroughly. Remove any greens and discard. Cut off each end and discard. Cut each carrot in half.
3. Process the pineapple and carrots through juicer.
4. For kids under 6 years of age: dilute with 1/4 cup water.
5. Pour juice into cup, over ice if desired.
6. Encourage your child to drink the juice immediately in order to benefit from all the nutrients. Any remaining juice can be refrigerated for up 48 hours, in an airtight, opaque container as to not be exposed to light, heat, or air due to risk of oxidation and loss of nutrients.

Nutritional info: Calories: 69 Total Fat: 0g Total Carbohydrates: 19g Dietary Fiber: 3g Sugars: 25g Protein: 3g Sodium: 21mg

Juicing Regimen for Kids: Week Two - Day Six

Apple – Grape Juice

Juice prep to finish: 4 minutes

Difficulty: Easy

Yield: (2) 4 oz. (125ml) cup

Ingredients:

- 2 to 3 medium apples of choice, skinned and sliced (make sure all seeds are removed)
- 2 to 4 cups grapes of choice, any stems removed
- 3/4 cup filtered water, to dilute (for kids under the age of 6)
- Ice, optional

Instructions:

1. Wash and skin the apple. Cut into slices and make sure all seeds are removed.
2. Wash grapes and make sure all stems are removed.
3. Process the apple slices and grapes through juicer.
4. For kids under 6 years of age: dilute with 3/4 cup water.
5. Pour juice into cup, over ice if desired.
6. Encourage your child to drink the juice immediately in order to benefit from all the nutrients. Any remaining juice can be refrigerated for up 48 hours, in an airtight, opaque container as to not be exposed to light, heat, or air due to risk of oxidation and loss of nutrients.

Nutritional info: Calories: 98 Total Fat: 0g Total Carbohydrates: 22g Dietary Fiber: 6g Sugars: 28g Protein: 2g Sodium: 4mg

Juicing Regimen for Kids: Week Two - Day Seven

Strawberry - Pineapple Juice

Juice prep to finish: 4 minutes

Difficulty: Easy

Yield: (2) 4 oz. (125ml) cups

Ingredients:

- 2 cups strawberries, stems removed, ends chopped off and discarded
- 2 to 4 cups of pineapple, cut into chunks
- ¼ cup filtered water, to dilute (for kids under the age of 6)
- Ice, optional

Instructions:

1. Remove all stems and leaves from strawberries and discard. Wash berries well. Chop off ends and discard.
2. Remove the rind and cut the pineapple into sections and then chunks until you have 2 to 4 cups of pineapple pieces.
3. Process the pineapple pieces and strawberries through juicer.
4. For kids under 6 years of age: Dilute with 1/4 cup water.
5. Pour juice into cup, over ice if desired.
6. Encourage your child to drink the juice immediately in order to benefit from all the nutrients. Any remaining juice can be refrigerated for up 48 hours, in an airtight, opaque container as to not be exposed to light, heat, or air due to risk of oxidation and loss of nutrients.

Nutritional info: Calories: 68 Total Fat: 0g Total Carbohydrates: 19g Dietary Fiber: 4g Sugars: 24g Protein: 3g Sodium: 5mg

Juicing Regimen for Kids – Week Three

Week three's recipes combine three different types of fruits or vegetables. The recipes are still very simple and your child should do fairly well with accepting these juices.

Juicing Regimen for Kids: Week Three - Day One

Grapefruity Glitz

Juice prep to finish: 6 minutes

Difficulty: Easy

Yield: (2) 4 oz. (125ml) cups

Ingredients:

- 1 large cucumber, with skin
- 1½ to 2 oranges, peeled and sectioned
- 1 grapefruit, peeled and sectioned
- ¼ cup filtered water, to dilute (for kids under the age of 6)
- Ice, optional

Instructions:

1. Scrub the cucumber, and cut into long slices. Leave the skin on.
2. Peel oranges and section. Peel grapefruit and section.
3. Process the cucumber, orange, and grapefruit through juicer.
4. For kids under 6 years of age: dilute with 1/4 cup water.
5. Pour juice into cup, over ice if desired.
6. Encourage your child to drink the juice immediately in order to benefit from all the nutrients. Any remaining juice can be refrigerated for up 48 hours, in an airtight, opaque container as to not be exposed to light, heat, or air due to risk of oxidation and loss of nutrients.

Nutritional info: Calories: 102 Total Fat: 0g Total Carbohydrates: 11g Dietary Fiber: 7g Sugars: 27g Protein: 3g Sodium: 5mg

Juicing Regimen for Kids: Week Three - Day Two

Tutti Fruity

Juice prep to finish: 6 minutes

Difficulty: Easy

Yield: (2) 4 oz. (125ml) cups

Ingredients:

- 1 orange, peeled and sectioned
- 1 Golden Delicious apple, cored and sliced, seeds removed
- ½ banana, peeled and cut into long slices
- 1 kiwi, peeled
- ¼ cup filtered water, to dilute (for kids under the age of 6)
- Ice, optional

Instructions:

1. Prepare the fruit as directed above.
2. Process the orange through juicer.
3. Process the apple through juicer.
4. Process the kiwi through juicer.
5. Place the banana, juice, and ice in a blender. Blend until smooth.
6. For kids under 6 years of age: Dilute with 1/4 cup water.
7. Pour juice into cup, over ice if desired.
8. Encourage your child to drink the juice immediately in order to benefit from all the nutrients. Any remaining juice can be refrigerated for up 48 hours, in an airtight, opaque container as to not be exposed to light, heat, or air due to risk of oxidation and loss of nutrients.

Nutritional info: Calories: 102 Total Fat: 0g Total Carbohydrates: 11g Dietary Fiber: 7g Sugars: 38g Protein: 3g Sodium: 5mg

Juicing Regimen for Kids: Week Three - Day Three

Pine O' Broccoli

Juice prep to finish: 4 minutes

Difficulty: Easy

Yield: (2) 4 oz. (125ml) cups

Ingredients:

- 2 to 4 cups of pineapple, cut into chunks
- 4 broccoli spears
- 1 small bunch watercress
- 1/8 cup to 1/4 cup sparkling mineral water (to dilute)
- Ice, optional

Instructions:

1. Wash the broccoli.
2. Core and remove rind from pineapple, cut into chunks.
3. Process the broccoli, pineapple, and watercress through juicer.
4. Dilute the juice with 1/8 cup sparkling mineral water, to taste. Test the juice and add remaining 1/8 cup water, if needed, to taste.
5. Pour juice into cup, over ice if desired.
6. Encourage your child to drink the juice immediately in order to benefit from all the nutrients. Any remaining juice can be refrigerated for up 48 hours, in an airtight, opaque container as to not be exposed to light, heat, or air due to risk of oxidation and loss of nutrients.

Nutritional info: Calories: 92 Total Fat: 0g Total Carbohydrates: 31g Dietary Fiber: 6g Sugars: 25g Protein: 5g Sodium: 50mg

Juicing Regimen for Kids: Week Three - Day Four

Super Sipper!

Juice prep to finish: 5 minutes

Difficulty: Easy

Yield: (2) 4 oz. (125ml) cups

Ingredients:

- 2 cups seedless grapes, washed and stems removed
- 2 kiwis, peeled
- 2 cups strawberries, stems/leaves removed and ends chopped off
- 1/8 cup to 1/4 cup sparkling mineral water (to dilute)
- Ice, optional

Instructions:

1. Prepare fruit as directed above.
2. Process the grapes, kiwi, and strawberries through juicer.
3. Dilute the juice with 1/8 cup sparkling mineral water, to taste. Test the juice and add remaining 1/8 cup water, if needed, to taste.
4. Pour juice into cup, over ice if desired.
5. Encourage your child to drink the juice immediately in order to benefit from all the nutrients. Any remaining juice can be refrigerated for up 48 hours, in an airtight, opaque container as to not be exposed to light, heat, or air due to risk of oxidation and loss of nutrients.

Nutritional info: Calories: 118 Total Fat: 0g Total Carbohydrates: 24g Dietary Fiber: 2g Sugars: 32g Protein: 5g Sodium: 8mg

Juicing Regimen for Kids: Week Three - Day Five

Very Berry Banana

Juice prep to finish: 5 minutes

Difficulty: Easy

Yield: (2) 4 oz. (125ml) cups

Ingredients:

- 1 orange, peeled and sectioned
- 2 cups strawberries, stems/leaves removed and ends chopped off
- 1 banana, peeled and sliced
- ¼ cup filtered water, to dilute (for kids under the age of 6)
- Ice, optional

Instructions:

1. Prepare fruit as directed above.
2. Process the orange and strawberries through juicer.
3. Place the banana, juice, and ice in a blender, blend until smooth.
4. For kids under 6 years of age: dilute with 1/4 cup water.
5. Pour juice into cup.
6. Encourage your child to drink the juice immediately in order to benefit from all the nutrients. Any remaining juice can be refrigerated for up 48 hours, in an airtight, opaque container as to not be exposed to light, heat, or air due to risk of oxidation and loss of nutrients.

Nutritional info: Ⓨ Calories: 108 Ⓨ Total Fat: 0g Ⓨ Total Carbohydrates: 34g Ⓨ Dietary Fiber: 4g Ⓨ Sugars: 37g Ⓨ Protein: 6g Ⓨ Sodium: 12mg

Juicing Regimen for Kids: Week Three - Day Six

Lots O' Berries Juice

Juice prep to finish: 5 minutes

Difficulty: Easy

Yield: (2) 4 oz. (125ml) cups

Ingredients:

- ½ cup raspberries, washed
- ½ cup blueberries, washed
- ½ cup blackberries, washed
- ¼ cup filtered water, to dilute (for kids under the age of 6)
- Ice, optional

Instructions:

1. Prepare fruit as directed above.
2. Process the berries through juicer.
3. For kids under 6 years of age: dilute with 1/4 cup water.
4. Pour juice into cup. Pour over ice, if desired.
5. Encourage your child to drink the juice immediately in order to benefit from all the nutrients. Any remaining juice can be refrigerated for up 48 hours, in an airtight, opaque container as to not be exposed to light, heat, or air due to risk of oxidation and loss of nutrients.

Nutritional info: Calories: 78 Total Fat: 0g Total Carbohydrates: 32g Dietary Fiber: 2g Sugars: 31g Protein: 6g Sodium: 7mg

Juicing Regimen for Kids: Week Three - Day Seven

Mango Tango Melon

Juice prep to finish: 5 minutes

Difficulty: Easy

Yield: (2) 4 oz. (125ml) cups

Ingredients:

- ½ mango, cut into chunks
- 1 peach, pit removed and sliced
- 1 cup cantaloupe, cut into chunks
- ¼ cup filtered water, to dilute (for kids under the age of 6)
- Ice, optional

Instructions:

1. Prepare fruit as directed above.
2. Process the mango, peach slices, and cantaloupe through juicer.
3. For kids under 6 years of age: dilute with 1/4 cup water.
4. Pour juice into cup.
5. Encourage your child to drink the juice immediately in order to benefit from all the nutrients. Any remaining juice can be refrigerated for up 48 hours, in an airtight, opaque container as to not be exposed to light, heat, or air due to risk of oxidation and loss of nutrients.

Nutritional info: Ⴢ Calories: 119 Ⴢ Total Fat: 0g Ⴢ Total Carbohydrates: 32g Ⴢ Dietary Fiber: 6g Ⴢ Sugars: 38g Ⴢ Protein: 2g Ⴢ Sodium: 5mg

Juicing Regimen for Kids – Week Four

Week four's recipes combine three OR MORE different types of fruits or vegetables. The recipes are a bit more complicated, but are still very kid-friendly.

Juicing Regimen for Kids: Week Four - Day One

Grape-Strawberry Surprise

Juice prep to finish: 5 minutes

Difficulty: Easy

Yield: (2) 4 oz. (125ml) cups

Ingredients:

- Υ 1 cup seedless grapes, washed and stems removed
- Υ 1 peach, pit removed, and sliced
- Υ 1 cup strawberries, stems/leaves removed and ends chopped off
- Υ ¼ cup filtered water, to dilute (for kids under the age of 6)
- Υ Ice, optional

Instructions:

1. Prepare fruit as directed above.
2. Process the grapes, peach slices, and strawberries through juicer.
3. For kids under 6 years of age: dilute with 1/4 cup water.
4. Pour juice into cup. Pour over ice, if desired.
5. Encourage your child to drink the juice immediately in order to benefit from all the nutrients. Any remaining juice can be refrigerated for up 48 hours, in an airtight, opaque container as to not be exposed to light, heat, or air due to risk of oxidation and loss of nutrients.

Nutritional info: Υ Calories: 102 Υ Total Fat: 0g Υ Total Carbohydrates: 36g Υ Dietary Fiber: 4g Υ Sugars: 29g Υ Protein: 2g Υ Sodium: 4mg

Juicing Regimen for Kids: Week Four - Day Two

Banana Blueberry Juice

Juice prep to finish: 5 minutes

Difficulty: Easy

Yield: (2) 4 oz. (125ml) cups

Ingredients:

- 1 cup blueberries, washed
- 1 large banana, peeled and sliced
- 1 orange, peeled and sectioned
- ¼ cup filtered water, to dilute (for kids under the age of 6)
- Ice, optional

Instructions:

1. Prepare fruit as directed above.
2. Process the blueberries, banana, and orange sections through juicer.
3. For kids under 6 years of age, dilute with 1/4 cup water.
4. Pour juice into cup. Pour over ice, if desired.
5. Encourage your child to drink the juice immediately in order to benefit from all the nutrients. Any remaining juice can be refrigerated for up 48 hours, in an airtight, opaque container as to not be exposed to light, heat, or air due to risk of oxidation and loss of nutrients.

Nutritional info: Calories: 124 Total Fat: 0g Total Carbohydrates: 33g Dietary Fiber: 5g Sugars: 31g Protein: 5g Sodium: 4mg

Juicing Regimen for Kids: Week Four - Day Three

Citrus Green Juice

Juice prep to finish: 5 minutes

Difficulty: Easy

Yield: (2) 4 oz. (125ml) cups

Ingredients:

- 1 small handful of baby spinach, washed
- 2 sticks celery, ends chopped off and discarded; cut stalks into sections
- 2 oranges, peeled and sectioned
- ¼ cup filtered water, to dilute (for kids under the age of 6)
- Ice, optional

Instructions:

1. Prepare fruit and vegetables as directed above.
2. Process the spinach, celery, and orange sections through juicer.
3. For kids under 6 years of age: dilute with 1/4 cup water.
4. Pour juice into cup. Pour over ice, if desired.
5. Encourage your child to drink the juice immediately in order to benefit from all the nutrients. Any remaining juice can be refrigerated for up 48 hours, in an airtight, opaque container as to not be exposed to light, heat, or air due to risk of oxidation and loss of nutrients.

Nutritional info: Calories: 112 Total Fat: 0g Total Carbohydrates: 23g Dietary Fiber: 6g Sugars: 24g Protein: 4g Sodium: 8mg

Juicing Regimen for Kids: Week Four - Day Four

Rainbow Juice

Juice prep to finish: 5 minutes

Difficulty: Easy

Yield: (2) 4 oz. (125ml) cups

Ingredients:

- 1 cup raspberries, washed
- 1 cup strawberries, stems/leaves removed and ends chopped off
- 1 large banana, peeled and sliced
- 1 orange, peeled and sectioned
- ¼ cup filtered water, to dilute (for kids under the age of 6)
- 4 to 6 ice cubes

Instructions:

1. Prepare fruit as directed above.
2. Process the raspberries, strawberries, and orange sections through juicer.
3. Place the banana, processed juice, and ice into blender. Blend until smooth.
4. For kids under 6 years of age: dilute with 1/4 cup water.
5. Pour juice into cup.
6. Encourage your child to drink the juice immediately in order to benefit from all the nutrients. Any remaining juice can be refrigerated for up 48 hours, in an airtight, opaque container as to not be exposed to light, heat, or air due to risk of oxidation and loss of nutrients.

Nutritional info: Calories: 136 Total Fat: 0g Total Carbohydrates: 32g Dietary Fiber: 2g Sugars: 36g Protein: 3g Sodium: 6mg

Juicing Regimen for Kids: Week Four - Day Five

Blackberries and Cream

Juice prep to finish: 5 minutes

Difficulty: Easy

Yield: (2) 4 oz. (125ml) cups

Ingredients:

- 2 medium apples of choice, washed, skinned, and sliced (make sure all seeds are removed)
- 2 cups blackberries, washed
- ½ cup low-fat Greek or natural vanilla yogurt
- 1 tsp. softened and runny natural honey (use microwave to soften, if needed)
- ¼ cup filtered water, to dilute (for kids under the age of 6)
- 4 to 6 Ice cubes

Instructions:

1. Prepare fruit as directed above.
2. Process the apple slices and blackberries through juicer.
3. Pour juice into Blender. Add in yogurt, honey, and ice. Blend until smooth.
4. For kids under 6 years of age: dilute with 1/4 cup water.
5. Pour juice into cup.
6. Encourage your child to drink the juice immediately in order to benefit from all the nutrients. Any remaining juice can be refrigerated for up 48 hours, in an airtight, opaque container as to not be exposed to light, heat, or air due to risk of oxidation and loss of nutrients.

Nutritional info: Calories: 142 Total Fat: 0g Total Carbohydrates: 43g Dietary Fiber: 6g Sugars: 52g Protein: 7g Sodium: 78mg

Juicing Regimen for Kids: Week Four - Day Six

Veggie Delight

Juice prep to finish: 8 minutes

Difficulty: Easy

Yield: (2) 4 oz. (125ml) cups

Ingredients:

- 1 to 2 carrots, greens removed, ends chopped off and discarded
- 1 tomato, cut into slices
- 1/8 cabbage, cut into pieces
- 2 celery stalks, ends removed and cut in pieces
- ½ small bunch of broccoli florets, washed and pulled apart
- ¼ cup filtered water, to dilute (for kids under the age of 6)
- Ice, optional

Instructions:

1. Prepare vegetables as directed above.
2. Process each vegetable through juicer.
3. For kids under 6 years of age, dilute with 1/4 cup water.
4. Pour juice into cup. Pour over ice, if desired
5. Encourage your child to drink the juice immediately in order to benefit from all the nutrients. Any remaining juice can be refrigerated for up 48 hours, in an airtight, opaque container as to not be exposed to light, heat, or air due to risk of oxidation and loss of nutrients.

Nutritional info: Calories: 128 Total Fat: 0g Total Carbohydrates: 36g Dietary Fiber: 10g Sugars: 29g Protein: 5g Sodium: 24mg

Juicing Regimen for Kids: Week Four - Day Seven

Apple Mint Juice

Juice prep to finish: 8 minutes

Difficulty: Easy

Yield: (2) 4 oz. (125ml) cups

Ingredients:

- 2 celery stalks, ends removed and cut in pieces
- 2 medium apples of choice, washed, skinned, and sliced (make sure all seeds are removed)
- 4 sprigs fresh mint
- 1 lime, peeled and sliced
- ¼ cup filtered water, to dilute (for kids under the age of 6)
- Ice, optional

Instructions:

1. Prepare fruits and vegetables as directed above.
2. Process celery, apple, lime, and mint through juicer.
3. For kids under 6 years of age, dilute with 1/4 cup water.
4. Pour juice into cup. Pour over ice, if desired.
5. Encourage your child to drink the juice immediately in order to benefit from all the nutrients. Any remaining juice can be refrigerated for up 48 hours, in an airtight, opaque container as to not be exposed to light, heat, or air due to risk of oxidation and loss of nutrients.

Nutritional info: Calories: 78 Total Fat: 0g Total Carbohydrates: 21g Dietary Fiber: 3g Sugars: 29g Protein: 1g Sodium: 11mg

CHAPTER 7: KID-FRIENDLY JUICING RECIPES THAT HEAL

Recipes to Treat Common Childhood Ailments & Disorders

Fresh fruits and vegetables are famous for their healing properties. When kids are sick with the common colds or stomach viruses, the last thing they want to do is eat, but they are typically willing to sip on something cold. This is where juicing is a miracle worker! You are able to get your children to consume these healing fruits and vegetables without having to force or bribe them to eat.

There are juicing recipes out there to help prevent, alleviate symptoms of, or cure most illnesses and disorders. The following recipes are of a few juices that will help aid in the speedy recovery from many common childhood ailments or complaints, including:

- Common colds
- Cough and congestion
- Flu Virus
- Lack of focus and concentration
- Anxiety
- Weight problems
- Diarrhea, constipation, gas

Let's get started!

Juicing Recipes for Kids: Common Cold, Cough, and Congestion

Get Well Juice

Juice prep to finish: 4 minutes

Difficulty: Easy

Yield: (2) 4 oz. (125ml) cups

Ingredients:

- 2 oranges, peeled and sectioned
- 1 grapefruit, peeled and sectioned
- 1 lime, peeled and sliced
- ½ cup cranberries, washed
- ¼ cup filtered water, to dilute (for kids under the age of 6)
- Ice, optional

Instructions:

1. Prepare fruits as directed above.
2. Process orange, grapefruit, lime, and cranberries through juicer.
3. For kids under 6 years of age, dilute with 1/4 cup water.
4. Pour juice into cup. Pour over ice, if desired
5. Encourage your child to drink the juice immediately in order to benefit from all the nutrients. Any remaining juice can be refrigerated for up 48 hours, in an airtight, opaque container as to not be exposed to light, heat, or air due to risk of oxidation and loss of nutrients.

Nutritional info: Ⓨ Calories: 112 Ⓨ Total Fat: 0g Ⓨ Total Carbohydrates: 32g Ⓨ Dietary Fiber: 2g Ⓨ Sugars: 36g Ⓨ Protein: 0g Ⓨ Sodium: 8mg

Juicing Recipes for Kids: Common Cold, Cough, and Congestion

Chin Up! Juice

Juice prep to finish: 4 minutes

Difficulty: Easy

Yield: (2) 4 oz. (125ml) cups

Ingredients:

- 3 carrots, greens removed, ends chopped off and discarded
- 6 spinach leaves, washed and torn
- 1/8 garlic clove, peeled and sliced
- ½ lemon, peeled and sectioned
- 1/8 teaspoon cayenne pepper
- ¼ cup filtered water, to dilute (for kids under the age of 6)
- Ice, optional

Instructions:

1. Prepare produce as directed above.
2. Process carrots, spinach, garlic, and lemon through juicer.
3. Stir in 1/8 teaspoon cayenne pepper.
4. For kids under 6 years of age, dilute with 1/4 cup water.
5. Pour juice into cup. Pour over ice, if desired
6. Encourage your child to drink the juice immediately in order to benefit from all the nutrients. Any remaining juice can be refrigerated for up 48 hours, in an airtight, opaque container as to not be exposed to light, heat, or air due to risk of oxidation and loss of nutrients.

Nutritional info: Calories: 87 Total Fat: 0g Total Carbohydrates: 29g Dietary Fiber: 6g Sugars: 23g Protein: 0g Sodium: 10mg

Juicing Recipes for Kids: Immune Health

Celery-Broccoli Juice

Juice prep to finish: 4 minutes

Difficulty: Easy

Yield: (2) 4 oz. (125ml) cups

Ingredients:

- 1 stalk broccoli, washed
- 4 medium carrots, greens removed, ends chopped off and discarded
- 2 large stalks celery, washed and ends chopped off; stalks cut into sections
- ¼ cup filtered water, to dilute (for kids under the age of 6)
- Ice, optional

Instructions:

1. Prepare vegetables as directed above.
2. Process vegetables through juicer.
3. For kids under 6 years of age, dilute with 1/4 cup water.
4. Pour juice into cup. Pour over ice, if desired.
5. Encourage your child to drink the juice immediately in order to benefit from all the nutrients. Any remaining juice can be refrigerated for up 48 hours, in an airtight, opaque container as to not be exposed to light, heat, or air due to risk of oxidation and loss of nutrients.

Nutritional info: Calories: 58 ⅂ Total Fat: 0.5g ⅂ Total Carbohydrates: 18g ⅂ Dietary Fiber: 6g ⅂ Sugars: 8g ⅂ Protein: 3g ⅂ Sodium: 110mg

Juicing Recipes for Kids: Immune Health

Mint-Berry Juice

Juice prep to finish: 5 minutes

Difficulty: Easy

Yield: (2) 4 oz. (125ml) cups

Ingredients:

- Υ 2 cups blueberries, washed
- Υ 2 kiwis, peeled
- Υ 25 mint leaves, scrunched up into a tiny ball or rolled into a piece of lettuce (to simplify the juicing process)
- Υ 15 medium strawberries, washed, stems/leaves removed, ends chopped off
- Υ ¼ cup filtered water, to dilute (for kids under the age of 6)
- Υ Ice, optional

Instructions:

1. Prepare fruits and vegetables as directed above.
2. Process through juicer one type of produce at a time, the mint should be last.
3. For kids under 6 years of age, dilute with 1/4 cup water.
4. Pour juice into cup. Pour over ice, if desired.
5. Encourage your child to drink the juice immediately in order to benefit from all the nutrients. Any remaining juice can be refrigerated for up 48 hours, in an airtight, opaque container as to not be exposed to light, heat, or air due to risk of oxidation and loss of nutrients.

Nutritional info: Υ Calories: 116 Υ Total Fat: 1.3g Υ Total Carbohydrates: 34g Υ Dietary Fiber: 8g Υ Sugars: 25g Υ Protein: 2.5g Υ Sodium: 5mg

Juicing Recipes for Kids: Focus and Concentration

CocoBananaRama!

Juice prep to finish: 5 minutes

Difficulty: Intermediate

Yield: (2) 4 oz. cups

Ingredients:

- One banana
- One mango (seeded, stings and skin removed)
- 2 tablespoons fresh lemon
- ½ cup coconut milk
- 1 teaspoon wheat germ
- 1 cup crushed ice
- ¼ cup filtered water, to dilute (for kids under the age of 6)
- Shaved coconut, to garnish

Instructions:

1. In blender, blend banana and mango for 15 – 20 seconds.
2. Add lemon and wheat germ, blend 15 seconds.
3. Lastly, add ice to blender and blend an additional 15 – 30 seconds, or until well blended.
4. For kids under 6 years of age, dilute with 1/4 cup water.
5. Pour juice into cup. Pour over ice, if desired
6. Encourage your child to drink the juice immediately in order to benefit from all the nutrients. Any remaining juice can be refrigerated for up 48 hours, in an airtight, opaque container as to not be exposed to light, heat, or air due to risk of oxidation and loss of nutrients.

Nutritional info: Calories: 111 Total Fat 3g Total Carbohydrates 21g Dietary Fiber 4g Sugars 15g Protein 3g Sodium 14mg

Juicing Recipes for Kids: Focus and Concentration

Attention Grabber Grape Juice

Juice prep to finish: 5 minutes

Difficulty: Easy

Yield: (2) 4 oz. glass

Ingredients:

- 2 cups purple or black grapes
- 1 cup fresh, sliced strawberries – OR – 1 cup frozen strawberries, thawed
- 1 apple, cored and wedged
- 2 tablespoons ginseng powder (available at any health food store)
- ¼ cup filtered water, to dilute (for kids under the age of 6)
- Ice, optional

Instructions:

1. Cut and process apple to fit juicer's feed tube. Juice apple.
2. Next, process grapes and strawberries through juicer.
3. Pour juice into glass. Add ginseng powder and stir with spoon to ensure that all ingredients are very well blended.
4. For kids under 6 years of age, dilute with 1/4 cup water.
5. Pour juice into cup. Pour over ice, if desired.
6. Encourage your child to drink the juice immediately in order to benefit from all the nutrients. Any remaining juice can be refrigerated for up 48 hours, in an airtight, opaque container as to not be exposed to light, heat, or air due to risk of oxidation and loss of nutrients.

Nutritional info: Calories: 89 Total Fat 0g Total Carbohydrates 27g Dietary Fiber 3g Sugars 27g Protein 2g Sodium 3mg

Juicing Recipes for Kids: Stress and Anxiety

Smooth Sailing Celery Juice

Juice prep to finish: 5 minutes

Difficulty: Easy

Yield: (2) 4 oz. glass

Ingredients:

- 6 stalks celery, ends chopped off
- 1 tbsp. honey
- ¼ cup filtered water, to dilute (for kids under the age of 6)
- Ice, optional

Instructions:

1. Cut and process apple to fit juicer's feed tube. Juice apple.
2. Next, process grapes and strawberries through juicer.
3. Pour juice into glass. Add ginseng powder and stir with spoon to ensure that all ingredients are very well blended.
4. For kids under 6 years of age, dilute with 1/4 cup water.
5. Pour juice into cup. Pour over ice, if desired.
6. Encourage your child to drink the juice immediately in order to benefit from all the nutrients. Any remaining juice can be refrigerated for up 48 hours, in an airtight, opaque container as to not be exposed to light, heat, or air due to risk of oxidation and loss of nutrients.

Nutritional info: Y Calories: 32 Y Total Fat 0g Y Total Carbohydrates 9g Y Dietary Fiber 0.5g Y Sugars 8g Y Protein 0.5g Y Sodium 98mg

Juicing Recipes for Kids: Stress and Anxiety

Apple-Cucumber-Spinach Juice

Juice prep to finish: 5 minutes

Difficulty: Easy

Yield: (2) 4 oz. glass

Ingredients:

- ᛉ 2 to 3 medium apples of choice, skinned and sliced (make sure all seeds are removed)
- ᛉ 1 large cucumbers, with skin intact
- ᛉ 6 leaves baby spinach
- ᛉ ¼ cup filtered water, to dilute (for kids under the age of 6)
- ᛉ Ice, optional

Instructions:

1. Wash and skin the apple. Cut into slices and make sure all seeds are removed.
2. Wash cucumber thoroughly. Cut into sections, keeping skin intact.
3. Process apple and cucumber through juicer. Process spinach through juicer.
4. For kids under 6 years of age, dilute with 1/4 cup water.
5. Pour juice into cup. Pour over ice, if desired.
6. Encourage your child to drink the juice immediately in order to benefit from all the nutrients. Any remaining juice can be refrigerated for up 48 hours, in an airtight, opaque container as to not be exposed to light, heat, or air due to risk of oxidation and loss of nutrients.

Nutritional info: ᛉ Calories: 25 ᛉ Total Fat 0g ᛉ Total Carbohydrates 7g ᛉ Dietary Fiber 0.5g ᛉ Sugars 5g ᛉ Protein 2g ᛉ Sodium 60mg

Juicing Recipes for Kids: Weight Management

Watermelon Eruption

Juice prep to finish: 5 minutes

Difficulty: Easy

Yield: (2) 4 oz. glass

Ingredients:

- 1 cooking apple, unpeeled, cored, and quartered
- 1 cups watermelon chunks, peeled, and deseeded
- 3oz. broccoli florets, washed, and stems removed
- 1 handful watercress
- ¼ cup filtered water, to dilute (for kids under the age of 6)
- Ice, optional

Instructions:

1. Process cooking apple, watermelon chunks, broccoli florets, and watercress into juicer.
2. For kids under 6 years of age, dilute with 1/4 cup water.
3. Pour juice into cup. Pour over ice, if desired.
4. Encourage your child to drink the juice immediately in order to benefit from all the nutrients. Any remaining juice can be refrigerated for up 48 hours, in an airtight, opaque container as to not be exposed to light, heat, or air due to risk of oxidation and loss of nutrients.

Nutritional info: ▼ Calories: 78 ▼ Total Fat 2g ▼ Total Carbohydrates 16g ▼ Dietary Fiber 2g ▼ Sugars 25g ▼ Protein 1g ▼ Sodium 4mg

Juicing Recipes for Kids: Weight Management

Strawberry-Lime Sparkler

Juice prep to finish: 5 minutes

Difficulty: Easy

Yield: (2) 4 oz. glass

Ingredients:

- 4 oz. fresh strawberries, hulled - OR – frozen strawberries, thawed
- ½ lime, peeled and sectioned
- ½ cup (4 fl. oz.) soda water
- 1 teaspoon Ginseng powder (available anytime at any health food store)
- ¼ cup filtered water, to dilute (for kids under the age of 6)
- Ice, optional

Instructions:

1. In juicer, process strawberries. Then add the lime.
2. Add soda water. When well blended, add Ginseng powder.
3. For kids under 6 years of age, dilute with 1/4 cup water.
4. Pour juice into cup. Pour over ice, if desired.
5. Encourage your child to drink the juice immediately in order to benefit from all the nutrients. Any remaining juice can be refrigerated for up 48 hours, in an airtight, opaque container as to not be exposed to light, heat, or air due to risk of oxidation and loss of nutrients.

Nutritional info: Calories: 117 Total Fat 1.4g Total Carbohydrates 8g Dietary Fiber 1.9g Sugars 4g Protein 3g Sodium 8mg

Juicing Recipes for Kids: Diarrhea, Constipation, Gas

Blue Veggie Juice

Juice prep to finish: 5 minutes

Difficulty: Easy

Yield: (2) 4 oz. glass

Ingredients:

- Ⓨ 1 medium Granny Smith apple, cored/seeds removed and sliced
- Ⓨ 1 cup blueberries, washed
- Ⓨ 1 stalk broccoli, washed
- Ⓨ 6 large carrots, scrubbed, greens removed, ends chopped off
- Ⓨ ¼ cup filtered water, to dilute (for kids under the age of 6)
- Ⓨ Ice, optional

Instructions:

1. Prepare all produce as directed.
2. Process all produce through juicer.
3. For kids under 6 years of age, dilute with 1/4 cup water.
4. Pour juice into cup. Pour over ice, if desired.
5. Encourage your child to drink the juice immediately in order to benefit from all the nutrients. Any remaining juice can be refrigerated for up 48 hours, in an airtight, opaque container as to not be exposed to light, heat, or air due to risk of oxidation and loss of nutrients.

Nutritional info: Ⓨ Calories: 122 Ⓨ Total Fat 1g Ⓨ Total Carbohydrates 38g Ⓨ Dietary Fiber 2g Ⓨ Sugars 20g Ⓨ Protein 3g Ⓨ Sodium 110mg

Juicing Recipes for Kids: Diarrhea, Constipation, Gas

Tropical Juice

Juice prep to finish: 5 minutes

Difficulty: Easy

Yield: (2) 4 oz. glass

Ingredients:

- 2 medium peaches, washed and pits removed
- 2 medium pears, washed and cut into sections
- 1 cup pineapple, cut into chunks
- ¼ cup filtered water, to dilute (for kids under the age of 6)
- Ice, optional

Instructions:

1. Prepare fruits as directed.
2. Process peaches, pears, and pineapple through juicer.
3. For kids under 6 years of age, dilute with 1/4 cup water.
4. Pour juice into cup. Pour over ice, if desired
5. Encourage your child to drink the juice immediately in order to benefit from all the nutrients. Any remaining juice can be refrigerated for up 48 hours, in an airtight, opaque container as to not be exposed to light, heat, or air due to risk of oxidation and loss of nutrients.

Nutritional info: Calories: 105 Total Fat 1g Total Carbohydrates 45g Dietary Fiber 1g Sugars 35g Protein 2g Sodium 3mg

Made in the USA
Las Vegas, NV
19 July 2022

51852319R00077